Professionalism in
Physical Therapy

Professionalism in
Physical Therapy
History, Practice, & Development

Laura Lee Swisher, PT, PhD
School of Physical Therapy
University of South Florida
Tampa, Florida

Catherine G. Page, PT, MPH, PhD
School of Physical Therapy
University of South Florida
Tampa, Florida

ELSEVIER
SAUNDERS

ELSEVIER
SAUNDERS

11830 Westline Industrial Drive
St. Louis, Missouri 63146

PROFESSIONALISM IN PHYSICAL THERAPY: HISTORY, PRACTICE, &
DEVELOPMENT

Notice

Physical therapy is an ever-changing field. Standard safety precautions must be followed, but as new
research and clinical experience broaden our knowledge, changes in treatment and drug therapy may
become necessary or appropriate. Readers are advised to check the most current product information
provided by the manufacturer of each drug to be administered to verify the recommended dose, the
method and duration of administration, and contraindications. It is the responsibility of the licensed
prescriber, relying on experience and knowledge of the patient, to determine dosages and the best treatment for each individual patient. Neither the publisher nor the author assumes any liability for any
injury and/or damage to persons or property arising from this publication.

ISBN-13: 978-1-4160-0314-4
ISBN-10: 1-4160-0314-2

Acquisitions Editor: *Marion Waldman*
Developmental Editors: *Jacqui Merrell and Marjory I. Fraser*
Publishing Services Manager: *Linda McKinley*
Project Manager: *Gail Michaels*
Designer: *Amy Buxton*

Printed in the United States of America

Last digit is the print number: 9   8   7   6

This book is dedicated to those early physical therapists whose commitment and vision shaped the foundational concepts of professionalism in physical therapy and to our personal professional mentors, whose insight and professional generosity have contributed to our own professional development, which is the foundation of this text.

Reviewers

Lisa L. Dutton, PT, PhD
Associate Professor of Health Sciences
Dean, College of Health Professions
The University of Findlay
Findlay, Ohio

Matthew Hyland, PT, MPA, CSCS
President, Rye Physical Therapy and Rehabilitation
Rye, New York
Part-time Faculty, Member Mercy College Physical Therapy
Dobbs Ferry, New York

David Lake, PT, PhD
Department of Physical Therapy
Armstrong Atlantic University
Savannah, Georgia

George Maihafer, PT, PhD
Chair, School of Physical Therapy
Old Dominion University
Norfolk, Virginia

Anne Thompson, PT, EdD
Armstrong Atlantic University
Savannah, Georgia

Camilla M. Wilson, PT, PhD
Department of Physical Therapy
Wichita State University
Wichita, Kansas

Foreword

Professionalism in Physical Therapy: History, Practice, & Development is a comprehensive resource that explores the multifaceted professional roles and the professional development of the physical therapist in the United States. Drs. Swisher and Page challenged themselves to write a scholarly text to discuss professional roles and professional development, review the history of the profession within the health care systems in which it has operated, encourage us to think about our future in terms of our history, analyze the five roles of the physical therapists established in the *Guide to Physical Therapist Practice*, and identify principles and issues that should guide professional decision making in today's and tomorrow's practice arenas. They certainly have met their challenge in this most comprehensive resource.

The book begins with the historical perspective of the professional role of the physical therapist and takes us through the many definitions and models of *profession* and *professional*. The fluid concepts of individual and collective professionalism are stressed. The section on the history of the profession looks at our development as it occurred within the contexts of the social events, health care and legislative activities, and medical milestones from 1910 to the present. The book also includes a retrospective analysis of the evolution of ethics within the profession and a discussion of the contemporary practice issues facing the profession, including the Doctor of Physical Therapy degree, specialist certification, direct access practice, physical therapist assistants, the *Guide to Physical Therapist Practice*, and the political action activities of the American Physical Therapy Association (APTA).

The next five chapters of the book look at the five roles of the physical therapist that have been identified in the *Guide to Physical Therapist Practice*: patient/client manager, consultant, critical inquirer, educator, and administrator. The historical perspectives, the dimensions of these roles, and, when available, the ethical and legal issues concerning the roles are presented.

The chapter on patient/client management starts with the activities of evaluation, diagnosis, and prognosis and progresses to information on discharge planning and discontinuance of care. Outcomes, clinical decision making, referral and interpersonal relationships, and the technological advances that may affect patient/client management are explored.

The chapter on the physical therapist as consultant covers the roles in that arena, as well as the consulting process, consulting fees, the traits that make a good consultant, and the importance of trust in the consultative relationship.

The chapter on critical inquiry begins with a history of physical therapist involvement in this area and progresses to evidence-based medicine and outcomes research. The role of the staff physical therapist is examined in light of using research, publishing case reports, assessing new concepts and techniques, and serving as a research subject. Guidelines for critiquing research reports and assessing products and courses are also included in this chapter.

The chapter on the physical therapist as educator probes the many contemporary educational roles. These range from the physical therapists who provide instruction to patients/clients to tenured professors in institutions of higher education. Teaching opportunities in the clinic, continuing education courses, and the academic environment are all delineated. Theories of teaching and learning are also discussed.

The chapter on the physical therapist as administrator stresses the roles now common to all physical therapists in practice, including billing for services, documentation, and delegation and supervision of support personnel. This chapter includes theories of organization, management, and leadership. The varied responsibilities of first-line managers, midlevel managers, and chief executive officers are presented. The APTA Standards of Practice are some of the many figures provided.

Each of these five chapters finishes with interesting, thought-provoking case scenarios that challenge us to examine the roles of the physical therapist from professional and ethical perspectives.

The last part of this book explores the organizational, political, and cultural contexts of professionalism in the U.S. health care system and professional development, leadership, and exemplary practice as it pertains to the physical therapist. Projecting into the future, the authors examine the potential of the APTA to influence the individual, institutional/organizational, and societal realms of physical therapist practice.

The book is easy to read, contains many tables and figures, and at the end of each chapter includes questions and/or case scenarios for reflection on the content.

Drs. Swisher and Page are two exemplary teachers and mentors who have written an outstanding, very thorough book that I would recommend to all physical therapist practitioners and physical therapist students. It is always a pleasure to see how effectively background knowledge and skill come together to provide a truly unique resource.

Marilyn Moffat, PT, PhD, FAPTA, CSCS
Professor, Physical Therapy Department
New York University

Preface

We became interested in writing a text on professionalism in physical therapy because of the challenges we faced in teaching the depth and breadth of issues and skills that are included in this umbrella topic in physical therapy curricula. A major challenge in teaching this topic was the paucity of written resources to assist students in learning this material. Over the years in academics and clinical practice, we have seen many changes that have provoked questions about how the profession of physical therapy and our professional roles have been evolving.

We have been particularly interested in the impact of those changes on the day-to-day efforts of physical therapists. As faculty who are preparing graduates to make their efforts professional in the bigger context of the systems in which they work, understanding those changes and their impact becomes essential. This is especially important as the profession of physical therapy moves toward a doctoring profession.

Therefore we felt a need for a text that could provide a framework in which to organize content related to physical therapy as a profession, the professional roles of physical therapists, and their development as professionals. We hope that the text is of value to faculty who may be responsible for all or part of this content and to curriculum committees as they define this thread of content in their programs. We hope that students will become actively engaged in the content through the questions for reflection and scenarios in each chapter.

Physical therapists seeking an update on their profession, especially through the eyes of the American Physical Therapy Association's *Guide to Physical Therapist Practice*, will find this text valuable as a reflection on the profession's past as well as fuel for thought on current professional issues. Physical therapists who are beginning to explore opportunities beyond direct patient care will gather some insight into administration, consultation, and teaching.

The development of this text has been an enriching experience that has been a major part of our ongoing professional development. We have listened to our clinical colleagues about the challenges they face in providing quality patient care, we have listened to our fellow teachers discuss the challenges of teaching professionalism, and we have listened while our colleagues in many components of the American Physical Therapy Association debate important professional issues. This text is for them, from them. These interactions stimulated our thinking about professionalism, and we hope that the resulting text reflects the complexity of many issues that face physical therapists and the profession as a whole.

We thank all of the people—students, colleagues, patients—who have made us pause to think about some aspect of professionalism in physical therapy. We became prouder of the profession with each of these interactions because of the level of thoughtfulness and commitment to the profession that we have encountered. The willingness of these numerous people to solve the problems they identified and to look at the long-term, big picture made us confident and excited about the future of our profession.

Acknowledgments

This text on professionalism in physical therapy would not have been possible without the efforts of a number of people. We are especially grateful to Marion Waldman, Jacqui Merrell, Marjory I. Fraser, Gail Michaels, and Cynthia Mondgock. Their thoughts, motivational communications, and efforts were always professional, and we thank them for their assistance in making this text a reality.

Laura Lee Swisher
Catherine G. Page

Table of Contents

PART I   Historical Perspective and Professional Practice Issues, *01*

Chapter 1   Introduction: The Physical Therapist as Professional, *01*

Chapter 2   The History of a Profession, *23*

Chapter 3   Contemporary Practice Issues, *45*

PART II   The Five Roles of the Physical Therapist, *71*

Chapter 4   The Physical Therapist as Patient/Client Manager, *71*

Chapter 5   The Physical Therapist as Consultant, *93*

Chapter 6   The Physical Therapist as Critical Inquirer, *109*

Chapter 7   The Physical Therapist as Educator, *129*

Chapter 8   The Physical Therapist as Administrator, *149*

PART III   Professional Development and the Health Care System, *181*

Chapter 9   Professionalism in the Multiple Contexts of the U.S. Health Care System, *181*

Chapter 10   Professional Development, Competence, and Expertise, *193*

Chapter 11   Future Challenges in Physical Therapy, *209*

1

Introduction: The Physical Therapist as Professional

As much as we would like to think so, physical therapy is not yet completely recognized as a profession.

– Catherine Worthingham[1]

Before deciding on a definition of [physical therapy], physical therapists must decide whether they really want to be professional or just make believe they are by paying lip service to professionalism.

– Mary E. Kolb[2]

As a profession, we have arrived. We have defined our scope of practice. We have developed a unique body of knowledge. We are documenting the effectiveness of our outcomes. We adhere to a code of ethics. And we take responsibility for the well-being of patients and clients. True autonomy is the destination.

– Ben Massey, Jr.[3]

WHAT DOES PROFESSIONAL MEAN?

As Catherine Worthingham[1] observed in 1965, physical therapy has not always been considered a profession. In the 1966 Presidential Address to the American Physical Therapy Association (APTA), Mary Kolb described the definition of physical therapy in the *Dictionary of Occupational Titles* as narrow, technical, and obsolete; she called on physical therapists (PTs) to engage in a "reappraisal of the role of physical therapy and a more appropriate definition of the field."[2] Not until 35 years later could Massey[3] state that physical therapy had arrived as a profession.

Undoubtedly, most PTs currently in practice believe that they are professionals and would consider being called "unprofessional" an insult. However, even though most people use the term *professional* frequently in everyday conversation, its meaning may not be altogether clear or may differ among groups. For instance, athletes who are paid to compete are called "professionals" to distinguish them from amateur athletes. This use of the word clearly is in contrast to the ideas of Massey and Kolb. Indeed, the use of *profession* and *professional* varies so much that some have wondered aloud whether these words now mean anything at all.[4]

The concept of *profession* and *professional* has been the subject of vigorous scholarly debate spanning much of the twentieth century and continuing today. The rigor and length of the debates reflect the ambiguity and multiple meanings of these terms and their importance as societal concepts embodying the legitimate expectations of the public for certain attitudes and behaviors exhibited by professionals. Consumers who feel that they received inadequate or impersonal physical therapy services, for example, may complain that the PT "was not professional." Changes during the last 50 years in the way that professions are viewed have raised a number of important questions for professionals, scholars, and members of society. These questions include the following:

- Should an occupation be designated a profession on the basis of the possession of specific characteristics, the developmental process by which the profession as a whole has gained recognition and status by the public, or the power the profession is able to wield?
- Does being a professional still hold meaning? Have health care professionals been "deprofessionalized" by managed care and "deskilled" by bureaucratic control within organizations?
- Which is more important—the individual or the collective dimension of being a professional?
- Should medicine continue to be the paradigm for what it means to be a profession and a professional?
- Have professionals fulfilled their implied contract with society to be accountable and self-regulating?

Given such questions, exploring the meanings of *profession* and *professionals* in some depth is appropriate. This chapter defines related terms, provides some background on the concepts related to professionalism, discusses the evolution of PTs' ideas about professionalism in the United States, addresses specific attributes important to being a professional, and reflects on current and future issues in physical therapy professionalism.

Preliminary Definitions of Profession and Professional

The concept of *profession* is an ancient one that has roots in Greek and Roman times.[5] The early origins of the word are reflected in its Latin precursor *profiteor*, which means "to profess a belief." This root meaning suggests that professionals have historically been expected to have a sense of "calling," or vocation.[6] Although not everyone construes this calling as religious, society still expects professionals to exhibit dedication to their work and clients.

The following preliminary definitions provide a starting point for discussion: A profession is an occupation that is viewed by society as a profession on the basis of it characteristics, development, or power. Professionalism is the internalized conceptualization of expected professional obligations, attributes, interactions, attitudes, values, and role behaviors in relation to individual patients and clients and society as a whole. Professionalism may be collective (practiced by the profession as a whole) or individual.[7,8] *Individual professionalism* refers to the internalized beliefs of an individual member of a profession regarding professional obligations, attributes, interactions, attitudes, values, and role behaviors. *Individual professionalism* might also be called "professional role concept."

Sociological Perspective

Much literature has been devoted to the discussion of what it means to be a profession, especially in sociology. According to Ritzer,[9] sociological literature about the professions takes three approaches: structural, processual (or process), and power. The structural approach focuses on the static characteristics that an occupation must possess to be considered a profession. The process approach focuses on either the stages and developmental periods that an occupation must pass through or activities that its members must perform to achieve recognition as a profession. Those advocating the power approach believe that a profession's ability to obtain the political and social power to define its work is its most important characteristic. As Ritzer[9] notes, these three approaches are not mutually exclusive. Indeed, when defining the term *profession*, most people blend these approaches.

Structural Approach

Although Emile Durkheim[5] wrote about the positive functions of the professions as early as 1890, the structural approach to professions is most associated with Talcott Parsons,[10] the founder of the structural-functionalist school of sociology. In translating Max Weber's[11] work to English in the mid-1900s, Parsons became interested in the professions.[10] Weber (1864-1920) had delineated the characteristics of priests, which formed a foundation for later definitions of professionals, and had also discussed the link among professionalization, bureaucracy, and rationalization. Adherents of Parson's perspective believed that existing social structures were the result of the positive function they served within society.[10]

The work of Parsons precipitated a tremendous amount of work in sociology during the 1950s and 1960s focusing on the professions. Much of this scholarship attempted to further refine the characteristics of the of true professions, in contrast to "semiprofessions" or nonprofessions.[12] Although debate about the number and nature of these traits has been considerable, the classic definition of a profession includes at least four: a body of theoretical knowledge, some degree of professional autonomy, an ethic that the members enforce, and accountability to society (Box 1-1).

Processual Approach

The second sociological approach to professions places less emphasis on an abstract "ideal type" definition of characteristics of professions than on "professionalization"—the social processes or developmental stages through which occupations move to attain the power and status that professions have traditionally held in society.[9,15-17] Central to this perspective is the recognition that an occupation can enhance its autonomy and professional status through social and political actions. For example, legislation requiring a license to engage in a particular occupation stage partly represents public acknowledgment of the professional status attained by that occupation. In a classic article, Wilensky wondered about the "professionalization of everyone."[18]

Much of the sociological literature about professions has emphasized autonomy as the *sine qua non* of a profession. Those occupations with extensive autonomy in their work are considered "true professions"; those with less autonomy are either "semiprofessions" or not professions at all.[12] Moore[19] and Pavalko[20] built on the idea of autonomy as the defining attribute of professions in developing a continuum or hierarchy of professionalism. A hierarchical continuum of characteristics combines the structural and processual approaches to defining a profession.[9] Pavalko's continuum allows assessment of an occupation's level or stage of professionalization (Figure 1-1). Use of the continuum requires placing a mark along the line between occupation and profession that best represents where an occupation is in

Box **1-1   Characteristics of Professions Cited in the Literature**

Knowledge

- Broad, theoretical, generalized, systematic knowledge[13,14]
- Unique body of knowledge
- "Formal" knowledge[15]—knowledge that is "embodied and applied in and through the professional"[6]

Autonomy in professional decisions

- Autonomy from client[16,17]
- Autonomy from organizations or external parties[16,17]
- Autonomy in selecting colleagues

Authority

- Based on internal knowledge[13]
- Granted by society[15]
- Demonstrated by power and status in society
- Demonstrated by monetary and symbolic awards[14]

Education

- Extensive
- Skilled, technical, esoteric
- High standards for admission

Responsibility, Accountability, and Ethics

- Service orientation[14,15,19]
- Accountability and responsibility to society
- Formal code of ethics that members enforce
- Self-control of behavior through internalized professional ethic[14]
- Belief in self-regulation[16]
- Community interest more important than self-interest
- Fiduciary relationship and trustworthiness central[6]

Nature of work and decisions

- Important or essential to clients[16]
- Complex[14]
- Not routine[13]
- Not programmed[13]

Role and Identity

- Internally based on a sense of calling[6,13,17]
- Formed and driven by the professional group[13,17]
- Extending beyond the specific work situation[13]

---

the process of professionalization. Writing in 1970, Pavalko[20] described both pharmacy and occupational therapy as incompletely professionalized or "marginalized professions" at that time.

Power Approach

Although the earliest literature from the structural perspective emphasized the positive functions of the professions, discussion began to shift to the negative aspects of

Dimensions	Occupation		Profession
1. Theory, intellectual technique	Absent	——————————————	Present
2. Relevance to social values	Not relevant	——————————————	Relevant
3. Training period	A Short	——————————————	Long
	B Non-specialized	——————————————	Specialized
	C Involves things	——————————————	Involves symbols
	D Subculture unimportant	——————————————	Subculture important
4. Motivation	Self-interest	——————————————	Service
5. Autonomy	Absent	——————————————	Present
6. Commitment	Short term	——————————————	Long term
7. Sense of community	Low	——————————————	High
8. Code of ethics	Undeveloped	——————————————	Highly developed

Figure 1-1. Pavalko's occupation to profession continuum. *(From Pavalko RM. Sociology of occupations and professions. Itaska, Ill, 1971, FE Peacock Publishers, p. 26.)*

professions by the 1960s and 1970s. This academic shift toward analysis of the use and abuse of power by the professions was accompanied by changes in public opinion regarding the professions. Scholars and members of the public criticized the professions for setting up economic monopolies, using political power for self-interest, and focusing on professional autonomy and self-governance without consideration of the public welfare.[21] The requirement for licensure is one strategy for using political power to create an economic monopoly and decrease competition for members of a particular profession.

AUTONOMY, SELF-REGULATION OF ETHICAL STANDARDS, AND ACCOUNTABILITY

Whether a profession is defined by its characteristics, stage of evolution, or power, several qualities of professions have historically been held in high regard: autonomy, ethical standards, and accountability.

Autonomy

As the previous section suggests, autonomy in making professional judgments is a "litmus test" for professions. *Autonomy* can be defined as the "extent to which [a profession] or an individual feels freedom and independence in his/her role."[22] Some writers clarify that this includes freedom from clients (those outside the profession) and the organization that employs the professional.[16] Historically, those occupations whose members have had high autonomy in decision making and high degrees of control over their work have been considered true professions;

occupations whose members enjoyed less autonomy in decision making and less control over their work were relegated to being semiprofessions,[12] paraprofessions, or nonprofessions.

The shift toward managed care during the 1980s had a major impact on concepts of professions and professionalism. Managed care placed significant administrative restrictions on the decisions made by health care professionals. Many medical professionals perceived this loss of autonomy as a loss of professional status, or "deprofessionalization,"[23] because they were no longer able to freely make decisions based on their expertise and specialized training. As Reed and Evans described it, "Because of the crucial link between autonomy and professionalism, when considerable slippage in a profession's autonomy occurs, as it has in medicine, the possibility of deprofessionalization becomes more tangible."[23] Despite these negative effects, these changes have also stimulated medical professionals to reexamine concepts of professionalism. Within medicine, Stevens called for "reinventing professionalism"[24] and Sullivan pointed to the need for "civic professionalism."[25]

Whether PTs have enough autonomy in their work to be considered professionals has also been a subject of considerable discussion and debate. Until recently, the tendency has been to view physical therapy as an occupation in the process of professionalization but not yet fully recognized as a profession. However, many PTs have experienced significant increases in their autonomy over the last 20 years. One measure of professional autonomy is access to PTs without physician referral. In 1985, only 7 states allowed direct access of patients to PTs. By 2002, 35 states permitted direct access and 48 states allowed PTs to perform initial evaluations without referrals.[26]

The APTA has established the goal of "autonomous practice" as one of its priorities, delineated in its Vision 2020 statement: "Physical therapists will be practitioners of choice in clients' health networks and will hold all privileges of autonomous practice."[27] This raises the question of what is meant by "autonomous practice." The APTA Board of Directors has developed a position statement to define this term (Box 1-2).[28]

Use of APTA criteria to evaluate the level of autonomy exercised by PTs would undoubtedly result in enormous variation by state, practice, setting, and specific organization. Almost every PT exercises and acts on professional judgment, but few PTs have privileges to refer patients directly for diagnostic tests. At the same time, managed care and other third-party payers have imposed restrictions on most health care services, including physical therapy. Organizational constraints also may limit autonomy. For example, even in states that permit direct access, organizational policies may require a referral for physical therapy services because many third-party payers require a referral for reimbursement.

For much of physical therapy's history, PTs have worked under the supervision of or through referral from physicians. Given the importance assigned to autonomy in the process of professionalization, only within the last several decades has physical therapy approached what some would define as full professional status. Ironically, PTs have attained increased legal autonomy through direct access in most states while simultaneously experiencing decreased autonomy through the administrative constraints of managed care.

To many PTs the emphasis on autonomy seems out of touch with a health care environment that is characterized by interdisciplinary teamwork and collaboration. Jules Rothstein[29,30] suggests that autonomy is a misnomer for the type of independence that PTs desire[29]:

Box 1-2   APTA BOARD OF DIRECTORS' POSITION ON AUTONOMOUS PHYSICAL THERAPIST PRACTICE

It is the position of the APTA Board of Directors that:

Autonomous physical therapist practice is characterized by independent, self-determined professional judgment and action. Physical therapists have the capability, ability and responsibility to exercise professional judgment within their scope of practice and to professionally act on that judgment.

Privileges of Autonomous Practice in 2020

Each of these elements includes two overarching concepts: recognition of and respect for physical therapists as the practitioners of choice, and recognition of and respect for the education, experience, and expertise of physical therapists in their professional scope of practice.

1. *Direct and unrestricted access:* The physical therapist has the professional capability and ability to provide to all individuals the physical therapy services they choose without legal, regulatory, or payer restrictions.
2. *Professional ability to refer to other health care providers:* The physical therapist has the professional capability and ability to refer to others in the health care system for identified or possible medical needs beyond the scope of physical therapist practice.
3. *Professional ability to refer to other professionals:* The physical therapist has the professional capability and ability to refer to other professionals for identified patient/client needs beyond the score of physical therapist practice.
4. *Professional ability to refer for diagnostic tests:* The physical therapist has the professional capability and ability to refer for diagnostic tests that would clarify the patient/client situation and enhance the provision of physical therapy services.

From the American Physical Therapy Association. *Autonomous Physical Therapist Practice: Definitions and Privileges.* (BOD 03-03-12-28.) Available at http://www.apta.org/http://www.apta.org/AM/Template.cfm?Section=Search& template=/CM/HTMLDisplay.cfm&ContentID=13420. Accessed September 30, 2004. This material is copyrighted, and any further reproduction or distribution is prohibited.

> It's not really autonomy that we as a profession seek. . . . We seek *unfettered practice* that allows us to use our skills, knowledge, and compassion to our maximum potential. On behalf of patients and clients, we seek *unfettered access* to our services, free from unnecessarily restrictive laws and reimbursement policies. Like those we serve, we want to remove barriers.

In Rothstein's opinion, "interdependence is not a sign of weakness. Interdependence is a badge that civilized people wear to reaffirm their humanity, their capacity for kindness—and their competence."[29]

He extended this line of thinking in a later editorial[30]:

> As I expressed in a previous Editor's note . . . I believe that our call for autonomous practice is a terrible mistake. In today's health care environment, no one is truly autonomous—nor should anyone want to be autonomous when we consider the meaning of the word. . . . "Autonomy" conveys arrogance. Our profession has developed a specialized definition of "autonomous" [see Box 1-2 of this chapter]—one that removes most of its noxious qualities and focuses instead on the attainment of professionalism and professional recognition—but few outside our profession will have the ability or time to find that out.

An implicit assumption in Rothstein's writing is that the doctorate in physical therapy (DPT) will play a pivotal role in promoting autonomous practice of PTs. However, the expectation is that the DPT will better prepare PTs for autonomous practice—the ability to make independent decisions—and the permission to exercise that decision making depends on direct access legislation and reimbursement policies. Meanwhile, several factors seem to negate the importance of autonomous practice even if all PTs achieve it. For instance, the vertical and horizontal integration of health care systems most likely will limit the need for independent practitioners in all health professions. As a rule, PTs are employees (as are many physicians) rather than self-employed, the ideal status for autonomous practice. Third-party payers and providers more often negotiate decisions about where, when, and how often a person receives physical therapy than patients and physical therapists do. This has an impact on autonomous practice. PTs may not gain more autonomy in decision making just because they have DPT degrees and patients have direct access to them. Health care systems must continue to control costs and manage quality; the way PTs can practice autonomously while contributing to those goals in the health care systems that employ them is not clear.

The obvious alternative for ensuring autonomy is for all PTs to be independent contractors, but whether health care systems are prepared to offer staff privileges to PTs remains to be seen. The managerial challenges of having individual PTs following their patients through their health care experiences from acute care to outpatient to home care may be difficult to overcome in a health care system that is committed to providing all required services for patients admitted to their systems. PTs employed by the health care system may have difficulty working alongside PTs who appear and disappear when patients from their autonomous practices are admitted and discharged from a hospital. Health care systems also may be reluctant for discharged patients needing outpatient physical therapy to receive that care in centers other than those of the health care system. Having consumers identify strongly with the services of a particular PT may also prove challenging unless they have chronic conditions that require services across years.

However, PTs in their one-on-one relationships with patients have had variable degrees of autonomy in decisions about direct patient care. Particularly as the referral relationship with physicians has moved from prescription to blanket referrals for evaluation and treatment, PTs have had a great deal of autonomy in establishing and modifying plans of care. PTs have gained the trust of physicians for autonomy at this level through the outcomes of care they have achieved and their interpersonal relationship skills with individual referring physicians. Regardless of the academic degree PTs hold and limits of the law, these skills likely will remain the key to autonomous practice and its concomitant independent, self-determined judgment and action.

Self-Regulation of Ethical Standards

A second important characteristic of professionals is ethical conduct and self-regulation. This includes the possession of a code of ethics and mechanisms that ensure members abide by the code's principles. The American Physiotherapy Association, the forerunner of the APTA, adopted its first code of ethics in 1935.[31] The first code identified four major ethics violations: making a diagnosis, offering a prognosis, advertising for patients, and criticizing the doctor or other co-workers.[31] Although development of a code of ethics can be one sign of movement toward professionalization, Purtilo notes that this first attempt was not necessarily a success in this regard[32]:

Declaring a document a code of ethics does not in itself assume that one *has* a code of ethics! Elsewhere I have shown that the early attempts of the American Physical Therapy Association to design a code of ethics was gallant in its intent though unsuccessful in its outcome: one can hardly judge this document's set of rules designed solely to show devotion and complete deference to the physician as being grounded in any specifically ethical standards, even in the 1930s. While serving as a guide for good etiquette befitting the young ladies of the time, and while serving some other important ends, nonetheless, it did not serve as an *ethical* guide (Purtilo, 1977). Clearly more than good intent is required in the development of a code of ethics.

From this perspective, a true code of ethics articulates some professional consensus about the ethical standards that should guide practice and serves as the collective ethical wisdom of the profession, a map on the road to high ethical standards.

Other writers emphasize that a code of ethics is meaningless unless its members live by its ideals and enforce its provisions. The obligation to enforce a code of ethics is also called *self-regulation* and is frequently framed in terms of an implied social contract. By this logic, professionals have a great deal of autonomy and freedom that enables them to serve the interests of their clients. In return for this freedom, society expects responsible behavior and action in the public interest. For example, society expects professionals to take action against incompetent colleagues and provide pro bono care for those who cannot afford professional services. Unfortunately, many professionals fail to live up to the high standards espoused by professional codes of ethics, and few professions have been successful in policing their own ranks for ethical breaches. Most state chapter ethics committees for physical therapy receive few ethical complaints and refer even fewer to the Ethics and Judicial Committee of the APTA.

Accountability of Professionals

The third important attribute of professionals is responsibility and accountability. Taken together, these terms mean that professionals have obligations and must "account" to the public for the discharge of these duties. Emanuel and Emanuel define accountability as "the process by which a party justifies its actions and policies"[33] and delineate three separate models of accountability: professional, political, and economic.[34] Each model of accountability has different domains, components, content areas, and procedures.

Although the ethical standards for most health care professionals focus on accountability to patients inherent in the fiduciary relationship,[34] PTs and other health care providers are actually accountable to many different parties: the patient, the health care organization, other professionals, the government, and third-party payers (Figure 1-2). PTs have particularly felt the pull of competing accountabilities under managed care. Morreim[35] has described these competing accountabilities as a "balancing act" in which health care providers must balance the patient's interests with fiscal accountability for the public good. In addition, the financial incentives for cost containment in managed care create inherent conflicts of interest between the interests of the patient and the provider.

According to Emanuel and Emanuel,[34] medicine has traditionally used a professional accountability model in which health care professionals establish and enforce standards of accountability through professional organizations. In their opinion, the professional model is outdated and inadequate for the managed care context

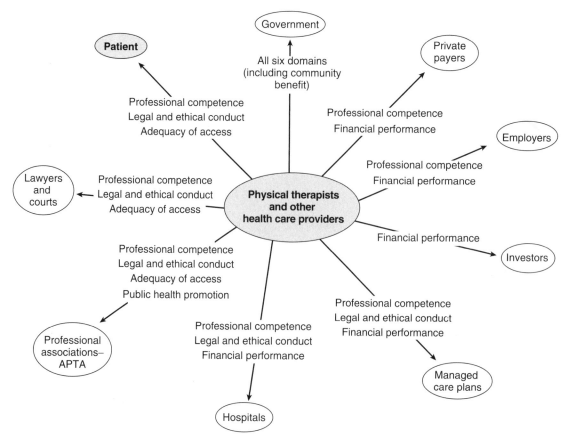

Figure 1-2. Accountability of physical therapists. *(Modified from Emanuel EJ, Emanual LL. What is accountability in health care? Ann Intern Med 1996;124:229-239, p. 229.)*

because it poorly addresses control of health care spending, one of the major goals of managed care. The difficulties of the professional model of accountability are further compounded by the decreasing numbers of PTs who actually belong to the professional association and the relative lack of success of all professions in self-regulation.

The views of Morreim and the Emanuels imply that different notions of professions and professional status may also have ramifications for the relationship between the physical therapy professional and the client. Ozar[36,37] developed three different models of professionalism to describe medicine and dentistry: commercial, guild, and interactive. These models of professionalism are also applicable to the work of the PT.

In the commercial model, professionalism is a commercial interchange in which physical therapy is a product or commodity and the therapist must compete with the patient and other professionals to sell services and maximize profit. Any duties of the therapist toward the patient are based on contractual agreements. In this model, professional associations exist to promote common business interests (Table 1-1).

In the guild model, the profession is the transmitter of expertise, competence, and moral standards. The PT functions in a paternalistic role, providing services to a patient who is the uninformed, passive recipient of professional expertise.

Table 1-1 | **Ozar's Models of Professionalism as Applied to Physical Therapy**

	Commercial	*Guild*	*Interactive (Ideal)*
Dominant concern	Maximizing profits	Advancing the profession as a service to benefit patients	Shared decision making by moral equals
Nature of PT's services	Commercial enterprise, commodity	Privilege	Expertise brought to interaction of moral equals
Role of PT	Salesperson	Expert, a representative of the profession	Moral equal, partner in decision-making
Role of client	Consumer	Passive recipient of expert knowledge	Moral equal, partner in decision-making
PT-client relationship	Competitors in self-interest	Paternalism demonstrated toward client, which may compromise client's autonomy	Mutual dialog in partnership of moral equals, each with different functions; autonomy of client valued highly
Criteria for determining PT intervention	Services client can afford and client's desires	Needs of client as determined by expert judgment of PT	Needs of client as determined through dialog
Relationship with other PTs	Competitors	Colleagues	Interaction of equals
Nature of professional associations (e.g., APTA)	Political action, public relations, and lobbying on behalf of shared business interests of members	Guardians of knowledge and skills	Partnerships of equals in dialog with the community, attempting to improve care
Derivation of obligations	Contractual agreements between client and therapist	Membership in the profession, which includes obligations to clients and colleagues; focus is on needs of client	Relationship with community, which bestows standing as a professional
Role of professional education	Marketplace for selling knowledge	Transformation of student into an expert, initiation into the guild	Provision of knowledge, although the community bestows professional status

Developed by LL Swisher from ideas of Ozar DT, Patient's autonomy: Three models of the professional-lay relationship in medicine. *Theor Med 1984;5(1):61-68; and Ozar DT,* Three models of professionalism and professional obligation in dentistry. *J Am Dent Assoc 1985; 110:173-177.*
PT, *Physical therapist;* APTA, *American Physical Therapy Association.*

Ozar believes that a third model, the interactive model, is the ideal model of the professional relationship. This model avoids the negative aspects of both the commercial and guild models, with therapists and patients interacting as moral equals in a relationship in which each person has a different function. Because the community has given professional status, the PT is obligated to care for the patient in need. The context for professional activity is construed as one of interaction between the PT and the community.[36,37] Bellner has argued that the interactive model of professionalism is most appropriate for occupational therapists and PTs because of its emphasis on "enhancing and supporting the patient's capacity to make choices."[38]

Although the meaning of the terms *profession* and *professionalism* continue to be subject to debate—with no general agreement among scholars, professionals, or the public as to whether a profession should be defined on the basis of its characteristics, the process of professionalization, or its power—the concept of the profession continues to hold some importance among members of society who expect professionals to provide professional expertise, have the freedom to act on their clients' behalf, be guided by ethical principles, and to demonstrate accountability in their actions. The various models provide opportunities to advance discussion of this important topic by clarifying which perspective of "profession" is the most critical.

PHYSICAL THERAPY AND CONCEPTS OF PROFESSIONALISM

Generally speaking, since its early years physical therapy's efforts to professionalize have concentrated on gaining increased autonomy, building a case for its expertise through improving education and scholarship, gaining public recognition, and enhancing political power through lobbying efforts. Especially from 1960 to 1990, PTs wondered whether physical therapy was a profession and were concerned with the public image of physical therapy (Box 1-3).

During this same period, physical therapy was especially concerned with the appropriate degree to offer, evidenced by several decades of debate about the move from the baccalaureate degree to the master's degree, followed by additional debate about the shift to the DPT degree. By the time the Commission on Accreditation established the master's degree as mandatory for all educational programs during the 1990s, most therapists realized that the DPT would eventually supersede this requirement. The following quotation from the APTA website illustrates how the physical therapy profession in the United States is working to accomplish further professionalization[45]:

> The rationale for awarding the DPT is based on at least four factors, among others: (1) the level of practice inherent to the patient/client management model in the *Guide to Physical Therapist Practice* requires considerable breadth and depth in educational preparation, a breadth and depth not easily acquired within the time constraints of the typical MPT [Master's in Physical Therapy] program; (2) societal expectations that the fully autonomous healthcare practitioner with a scope of practice consistent with the *Guide to Physical Therapist Practice* be a clinical doctor; (3) the realization of the profession's goals in the coming decades, including direct access, "physician status" for reimbursement purposes, and clinical competence consistent with the preferred outcomes of evidence-based practice, will require that practitioners possess the clinical doctorate (consistent with medicine, osteopathy, dentistry, veterinary medicine, optometry, and podiatry); and (4) many existing professional (entry-level) MPT programs already meet the requirements for the clinical doctorate; in such cases, the graduate of a professional (entry-level) MPT program is denied the degree most appropriate to the program of study.

Box 1-3   Professionalism as Described in the Physical Therapy Literature: 1935 to 1986

Miles-Tapping (1986)[39]	Medical dominance through subordination, limitation, and exclusion is rooted in the medical model of health care that allows physicians to define what counts as evidence and knowledge. "As long as physiotherapists base their understanding of disease and therapy on a medical model, cooperating and coordinating with doctors in their work, their profession will remain a dominated paramedical profession."[39]
Luna-Massey and Smyle (1984)[40]	Professionalism equals "strong motivation, established representative organization, a specialized body of knowledge, evaluative skills, and autonomy of judgment."[40] These criteria, established by Moore,[19] are listed in ascending order of importance. When California consumers used the criteria as a basis for evaluation, they found no significant difference in professional image between PTs and physicians.
Silva, Clark, and Raymond (1980)[41]	Using Moore's five criteria,[19] California physicians rated PTs lower on evaluative skills and autonomy than on other criteria. Family physicians rated PTs higher on professional image than did neurosurgeons or orthopedists.
Schlink, Kling, and Shepard (1978)[42]	California PTs' higher internal image conflicted with lower external professional image thought by PTs to be held by physicians and the public.
Dunkel (1974)[43]	Professionalism equals competence, concern, and a sense of responsibility.
	Physician's attitudes toward professional performance of PTs in Arkansas were rated.
Senters (1972)[44]	Professionalization equals "process of development toward an *ideal type*, the profession."[44]
	Physical therapy is "moderately professionalized."
Kolb (1960)[2]	Professionalism equals service orientation, theoretical knowledge, and autonomy.
	"Before deciding on a definition of [physical therapy], physical therapists must decide whether they really want to be professional or just make believe they are by paying lip service to professionalism."[2]
APTA (1935)[31]	In the first published code of ethics, professionalism is defined as etiquette and appropriate deference to authorities.

PT, Physical therapist; *APTA*, American Physical Therapy Association.

As indicated by this statement, the DPT degree links various aspects of professionalization: autonomy, attainment of adequate power, and status. The perception is that the DPT will enhance professionalization, enabling physical therapy to enjoy the professional status and power of other professions.

From 1990 to 2003, physical therapy scholars appeared to move away from the more general concepts of profession in an attempt to define the important attributes and behaviors of professionalism unique to physical therapy (Box 1-4). This coincided with a renewal in interest in professionalism in medicine stimulated in part by the perceived deprofessionalization resulting from managed care and increasingly negative societal views about professionals.

Box **1-4**   PROFESSIONALISM AS DESCRIBED IN THE PHYSICAL THERAPY LITERATURE: 1990 TO 2003

Swisher, Beckstead, and Bebeau (2004)[46]	Professionalism is a blend of autonomy, authority, agency, and responsibility. Factor analysis of results of the Professional Role Orientation Inventory.
APTA (2003)[47]	The seven core values of professionalism are defined as accountability, altruism, compassion/caring, excellence, integrity, professional duty, and social responsibility.
Jette and Portney (2003)[48]	Construct validation of the generic abilities cited by May et al.[53] identifies seven factors: professionalism, critical thinking, professional development, communication management, personal balance, interpersonal skills, and working relationships.
MacDonald et al. (2001)[49]	Consensus is found among students (n = 4), clinical instructors (n =3), and faculty (n = 2) on key professional behaviors: communication, adherence to legal and ethical codes of practice, respect, sensitive practice, lifelong learning, evidence-based practice, client-centered practice, critical thinking, accountability, and professional image.
Bellner (1999)[38]	Responsibility, an inherently relational concept, is posited as a central feature of professionalism. Bellner recommends that therapists embrace the interactive model.
Lopopolo (1999, 2001)[50,51]	Acute care clinical managers report that physical therapists' level of professionalism increased during hospital restructuring; fewer than one fourth report that it decreased.
Threlkeld, Jensen, and Royeen (1999)[52]	These researchers use the grounded theory model of professions, to analyze the DPT degree. The DPT is framed as the vehicle by which PTs attain appropriate professional status, identity, and outcomes.
May et al. (1995)[53]	Professionalism is included as one of 10 generic abilities: commitment to learning, interpersonal skills, communication skills, effective use of time and resources, use of constructive feedback, problem solving, professionalism, responsibility, critical thinking, and stress management. *Professionalism* is defined as "the ability to exhibit appropriate professional conduct and to represent the profession effectively."[53]
Hart et al. (1990)[54]	Professionalism equals esoteric knowledge, a service ethic, and autonomy in performing tasks. Physical therapy is in the process of professionalization. Level of professional involvement does not depend on the use of complex procedures, but PTs who are more professionally involved are more likely to receive referrals that require such complex procedures.

APTA, American Physical Therapy Association; *DPT*, Doctor of Physical Therapy; *PT*, physical therapist.

The scholarship on professionalism and the political actions of the APTA are consistent with the developmental stages identified as crucial to the professionalization of an occupation. Perhaps, physical therapy is taking its last steps toward professionalization.

INDIVIDUAL PROFESSIONALISM—PROFESSIONALISM WITHOUT PROFESSIONS?

Thus far, this discussion has focused primarily on collective professionalism. Given the level of disagreement about the importance of professions and concerns about whether professionals are living up to professional ideals, reflection on the personal meaning of professionalism is crucial for every professional. Society and individual patients will continue to have high expectations for professionals. Kultgen has proposed that society stop making distinctions between occupations and focus more on desirable attributes in individual workers, creating a situation that he calls "professionalism without professions."[5] This proposal would, he argues, preserve the positive aspects of professionalism without carrying forward its negative aspects.

Regardless of whether Kultgen's proposal is accepted, each professional frames professionalism uniquely because of differing emphases on each of the many dimensions of professionalism (authority, autonomy, responsibility, expert judgment, accountability, and ethical ideal). Relative emphasis on these dimensions brings some PTs closer to the commercial model, whereas others are closer to the guild or interactive model of professionalism. Some within medicine have called for a renewal of "civic professionalism"[25] as yet another model. Such an undertaking would require PTs to examine their implicit contract with society, collectively as a profession and individually as professionals.

Writing an individual or a collective oath can be a vehicle for reflection on a personal model of individual professionalism. The issue of whether PTs should take an oath similar to the Hippocratic Oath for physicians has been brought before the House of Delegates on several occasions. To date, PTs are not required to take an oath. Denise Wise[55] has researched proposals for an oath in physical therapy and summarized the history of these efforts in physical therapy:

> *History of an oath in PT:* The concept of an oath was first introduced to the House of Delegates in 1997 or 1998. In 2000, the position Oath for Physical Therapists (HOD 06-00-21-12) was passed. This position states: *It is the position of the APTA that:* The American Physical Therapy Association supports the use of an oath for physical therapists as part of a student's education and graduation from an accredited physical therapist education program or as an affirming statement for use by all physical therapists. In 1994, Dr. Donna El-Din[56] wrote the following in a guest editorial "Learning is an active process. The spoken word has power. Perhaps the learner rightly begins the process of validation in the professional commitment with the sound of the spoken word. Perhaps with . . . an oath."

Denise Wise[55] further stated the following:

> In 2000, it was decided to separate this position from a second RC that year that was ultimately withdrawn. This withdrawn RC was a model oath. Problems at that time included: not being clear it was a model oath and . . . a voluntary process. While there was support, there was also opposition. Since that time, several programs have continued to have an oath or affirming statement, with the knowledge that RC 06-00-21-12 was passed.

However, the process of formulating or revising an oath can be helpful in conceptualizing the obligations and commitments that a person or group believe are involved in professional life (Box 1-5).

FURTHER THOUGHTS

Neither individual nor collective professionalism is a static concept. History demonstrates that these concepts change and evolve in relation to societal need and opinions. Although professions and professionals no longer occupy a societal pedestal, members of the public continue to respect the judgments made by professionals and expect professionals to maintain high ethical standards. Some believe that society should abandon rigid distinctions between groups believed to be worthy of professional status and those that are not. In an environment of multiple meanings of the terms *profession* and *professional*, individual reflection on the personal meaning of these terms is especially important.

QUESTIONS FOR REFLECTION

1. Using Pavalko's continuum, how would you evaluate physical therapy's level of professionalization?
2. Using Pavalko's continuum, how would you evaluate your personal level of professionalism?
3. One criticism of professional codes of ethics is that society has no role in helping to write them.[5] What difference would it make if physical therapy involved the public in writing the *Code of Ethics*? As a member of the public, what changes would you recommend to the Guide for Professional Conduct?
4. Professions have also been criticized because of their lack of self-regulation, with few professionals being disciplined by the professional association. Members who are in danger of being disciplined can drop their membership, and the association has no authority to discipline nonmembers. Some states require all licensed PTs to abide by the code of ethics and ethical standards of the professional association. Do you support this action? Is this a type of self-regulation or is it public acknowledgment of lack of self-regulation?
5. Jules Rothstein[29-30] has suggested that physical therapy has placed too much emphasis on professional autonomy and that physical therapy should emphasize professionalism and interdependence. Do you agree? Why or why not?
6. Use Ozar's three models of professionalism (commercial, guild, interactive) to classify the model of professionalism used by some of the PTs in your community. How would clients and other colleagues classify these PTs' models of professionalism?
7. Bellner[38] suggests that the interactive model is the most appropriate model of professionalism for PTs. Do you agree with Bellner that the interactive model is most appropriate for physical therapy?
8. Ozar is candid in saying that he exaggerates the differences among his models to provide a clear distinction. As a result, both the commercial and guild models appear unattractive. Are realistic portrayals of the commercial and guild models acceptable for physical therapy?
9. Should PTs take an oath to demonstrate their commitment to professionalism?

Box 1-5   FOUR OATHS* FOR PHYSICAL THERAPISTS CORRELATED WITH PRINCIPLES OF THE CODE OF ETHICS

University of Southern California[†]	Wayne State University[‡]	New York University[§]	University of South Florida (2003)[‖]
I pledge to hold faithful to my responsibility as a physical therapist;	I solemnly and willingly state that I dedicate myself to the following:	In the presence of my colleagues, friends, families, and faculty, and in view of the honored profession into which I am entering, I solemnly and willingly dedicated myself to the following:	As a physical therapy professional, I embrace my responsibility and accountability to the individuals I serve, the community as a whole, and my profession. I believe that physical therapy is a calling to help the whole person—body, mind, and soul. As a physical therapist, I will strive not only to resolve movement disorders but prevent them, while inspiring others to reach beyond barriers and limitations. I commit myself to the following professional obligations and values:
To use the highest science and skills of my profession at all times; (5, 8)¶	I will practice physical therapy with compassion and patience. (1, 2, 10)	I will ethically practice physical therapy with compassion and patience, recognizing the potential vulnerabilities in my patients and clients, and will preserve their dignity and promote their health and well-being at all times. (1, 2, 10)	I will strive to approach each patient with compassion, encouragement, respect, and empathy. (1, 2, 11)
To exercise judgment to the highest degree of which I am capable when determining the treatment to be offered; (1, 2, 4, 6)	I will preserve and value the dignity of those who seek my care and will respect them, the choices they make, and the confidential nature of our relationship. (2, 3)	I will value the lives of those I serve through my concern and with respect for them and the confidential nature of our relationship. (2)	I will strive to provide an environment where patients can feel comfortable and accomplish the goals they set for themselves. (1-6, 10, 11)
To refrain from treatment when it will not benefit the patient; (2-4, 6, 8, 9, 11)	I will do no harm to another. (2-6, 8, 9, 11)	I will be humble. (2, 7)	I will strive to be a lifelong learner, seeking to advance my own knowledge as well as that of current and future colleagues. (4-6)
To always place the welfare of my patients above my own self-interest. (5-7)	I will promote health and well-being through the alleviation and prevention of impairments, functional limitations and disabilities due to illness or injury. (1, 2, 4, 6, 10)	I will recognize my limitations. (2, 4-6, 9, 11)	I will strive to achieve excellence in the practice of physical therapy. (1-11)
I pledge to uphold and preserve the rights and esteem of every person placed in my care; (2)	I dedicate myself to lifelong learning to augment and expand my knowledge and the profession through consultation, education, and research. (5)	I will continue to consult with my colleagues with which I may better serve my patients and clients and for the inspiration to expand and augment my education. (3-5, 11)	I will strive to relate to other professionals with respect and integrity in order to promote the best interests of the patient. I will uphold the highest ethical stands set forth by the profession. (1-6, 9)
To hold all confidences in trust; (2, 3)	I accept responsibility to assure those who seek physical therapy receive services that are proper, ethical, and just. (9)	I will share my knowledge freely with my colleagues and with those I serve. (1, 2, 6, 8)	I will respect diverse values, beliefs, and cultures. (11)
To exercise all aspects of my calling with dignity and honor. (1, 11)	I will not allow my judgment to be influenced by greed or unethical behavior. (7)	I will strive for an improved quality of life for all my patients and clients. (1, 2)	I will make these promises solemnly, freely, and upon my personal and professional honor.
I commit myself to the highest ideal of service, learning, and the pursuit of knowledge. (3-6, 8, 9, 11)	I expect the same from my colleagues. (6, 8, 9)	I will work to improve the practice of physical therapy so that all who seek	
These things I do swear.	Thus, with this oath, I freely accept the obligations and reward which accompany the practice of physical therapy.		

Continued

Box 1-5 **FOUR OATHS* FOR PHYSICAL THERAPISTS CORRELATED WITH PRINCIPLES OF THE CODE OF ETHICS—CONT'D**

University of Southern California†	Wayne State University‡	New York University§	University of South Florida (2003)‖
		physical therapy services will receive those which are proper, ethical, and just. (6, 8, 9) I will not allow my judgment regarding the practice of my profession to be influenced by greed or unethical behavior. (7) I will respect the rights of all persons. (1, 11) Thus, with this oath, I freely accept all of the obligations and the many rewards which will accompany my practice of physical therapy.	

Modified from Wise D. Oath compilation summary. Unpublished manuscript distributed by electronic mail, October 28, 2003.

*Those who submitted oaths were not always certain of their origin. Several of these oaths were thought to be based in part on an oath developed by Helen Hislop.

†Used with permission of James Gordon, PT, EdD.

‡Used with permission of Susan Ann Talley, PT, MA.

§Used with permission of Marilyn Moffat, PT, PhD, FAPTA.

‖Used with permission of Laura Lee Swisher, PT, PhD.

¶Numbers in parenthesis correspond to the following principles in the Code of Ethics established by the American Physical Therapy Association:

Principle 1: A physical therapist shall respect the rights and dignity of all individuals and shall provide compassionate care.

Principle 2: A physical therapist shall act in a trustworthy manner towards patients/clients, and in all other aspects of physical therapy practice.

Principle 3: A physical therapist shall comply with laws and regulations governing physical therapy and shall strive to effect changes that benefit patients/clients.

Principle 4: A physical therapist shall exercise sound professional judgment.

Principle 5: A physical therapist shall achieve and maintain professional competence.

Principle 6: A physical therapist shall maintain and promote high standards for physical therapy practice, education, and research.

Principle 7: A physical therapist shall seek only such remuneration as is deserved and reasonable for physical therapy services.

Principle 8: A physical therapist shall provide and make available accurate and relevant information to patients/clients about their care and to the public about physical therapy services.

Principle 9: A physical therapist shall protect the public and profession from unethical, incompetent, and illegal acts.

Principle 10: A physical therapist shall endeavor to address the health needs of society.

Principle 11: A physical therapist shall respect the rights, knowledge, and skills of colleagues and other health care professionals.

10. How would you describe your own model of professionalism?
11. What effect will awarding the DPT have on the professionalism of PTs?

REFERENCES

1. Worthingham CA. Second Mary McMillan Lecture: Complementary functions and responsibilities in an emerging profession. *Phys Ther* 1965;45:935-939.
2. Kolb ME. 1966 APTA presidential address: The challenge of success. *Phys Ther* 1966;46:1157-1164.
3. Massey BF Jr. 2001 APTA presidential address: We have arrived! *Phys Ther* 2001;81:1830-3.
4. Larson MS. Professionalism: Rise and fall. *Int J Health Serv* 1979;9(04):607-627.
5. Kultgen J. *Ethics and professionalism*. Philadelphia: University of Pennsylvania Press; 1988.
6. Sokolowski R. The fiduciary relationship and the nature of the professions. In: Pellegrino ED, Veatch RM, Langan JP, editors. *Ethics, trust, and professions*. Washington, DC: Georgetown University Press; 1991. pp. 23-29.
7. Connelly JE. The other side of professionalism: Doctor-to-doctor. *Camb Q Healthc Ethics* 2003; 12(2): 178-183.
8. Swick HM. Toward a normative definition of medical professionalism. *Acad Med* 2000;75(6):612-616.
9. Ritzer G. Professionalization, bureaucratization and rationalization: The views of Max Weber. *Social Forces* 1975;53(4):627-634.
10. Latham SR. Medical professionalism: A Parsonian view. *Mt Sinai J Med* 2002;69(6):363-369.
11. Weber M. *Economy and society: An outline of interpretive sociology*. Roth G, Wittich C, editors; Fischoff E et al., translators. Berkeley: University of California Press; 1978.
12. Etzioni A, editor. *The semi-professions and their organization: Teachers, nurses, social workers*. New York: Free Press; 1969.
13. Elliott P. *The Sociology of the professions*. New York: Herdman and Herdman;1972.
14. Barber B. Some problems in the sociology of professions. In: Lynn KS, editor. *The Sociology of the Professions in America*. Boston: Houghton Mifflin; 1965.
15. Freidson E. *Professional powers: A study of the institutionalization of formal knowledge*. Chicago: University of Chicago Press; 1986.
16. Forsyth BF, Danisiewicz TJ. Toward a theory of professionalization. *Work Occupations* 1985;12(1): 59-76.
17. Hall RH. Professionalization and bureaucratization. *Am Sociol Rev* 1968;33(1):92-104.
18. Wilensky HL. The professionalization of everyone? *Am J Sociol* 1964;70(2):137-158.
19. Moore WE. *The professions: Roles and rules*. New York: Russell Sage Foundation; 1970.
20. Pavalko RM. *Sociology of occupations and professions*. Itaska, Ill: F.E. Peacock Publishers; 1971.
21. Freidson E. The theory of the professions: State of the art. In: Dingwall R, Lewis P, editors. *The sociology of the professions: Lawyers, doctors, and others*. New York: St. Martin's Press; 1983.
22. Bebeau MJ, Born DO, Ozar DT. The development of a professional role orientation inventory. *J Am Coll Dentists* 1993;60(2):27-33.
23. Reed RR, Evans D. The deprofessionalization of medicine. *JAMA* 1987;258(22):3279-3282.
24. Stevens RA. Themes in the history of medical professionalism. *Mt Sinai J Med* 2002;69(6):357-362.
25. Sullivan WM. What is left of professionalism after managed care? *Hastings Cent Rep* 1999;29(12):7-8.
26. Massey BF Jr. 2002 APTA presidential address: What's all the fuss about direct access? *Phys Ther* 2002;82:1120-1123.
27. American Physical Therapy Association. APTA vision sentence and vision statement for physical therapy 2020 [HOD 06-00-24-35]. Retrieved December 8, 2004 at http://www.apta.org/About/aptamissiongoals/visionstatement
28. American Physical Therapy Association. Autonomous Physical Therapist Practice: Definitions and Privileges. (BOD 03-03-12-28) Available at www.apta.org/Documents/Public/governance/bodPoliSec1.pdf. Accessed September 30, 2004.

29. Rothstein JM. Autonomy and dependency. *Phys Ther* 2002;82(8):750-751.

30. Rothstein JM. Autonomy or professionalism? *Phys Ther* 2003;83(3):206-207.

31. Purtilo RB. The American Physical Therapy Association's code of ethics: Its historical foundations. *Phys Ther* 1977;57:1001-1006.

32. Purtilo RB. Codes of ethics in physiotherapy: A retrospective view and look ahead. *Physiother Pract* 1987;3(1):28-34.

33. Emanuel EJ, Emanuel LL. Preserving community in health care. *J Health Polit Policy Law* 1997;22(1):147-184.

34. Emmanuel EJ, Emmanuel LL. What is accountability in health care? *Ann Int Med* 1996;124: 229-239.

35. Morreim EH. *Balancing act: The new medical ethics of medicine's new economics.* Washington, DC: Georgetown University Press; 1995.

36. Ozar DT. Patient's autonomy: Three models of the professional-lay relationship in medicine. *Theor Med* 1984;5(1):61-68.

37. Ozar DT. Three models of professionalism and professional obligation in dentistry. *J Am Dental Assoc* 1985;110:173-177.

38. Bellner AL. Senses of responsibility. A challenge for occupational and physical therapists in the context of ongoing professionalization. *Scand J Caring Sci* 1999;13(1):55-62.

39. Miles-Tapping C. Physiotherapy and medicine: Dominance and control? *Physiother Canada* 1986;37(5):290-293.

40. Luna-Massey P, Smyle L. Attitudes of consumers of physical therapy in California toward the professional image of physical therapists. *Phys Ther* 1982;62(3):309-314.

41. Silva DM, Clark SD, Raymond G. California physician's professional image of therapists. *Phys Ther* 1981;61(8):1152-1157.

42. Schlink M, Kling R, Shepard K. *An attitudinal assessment of the professional image of California physical therapists* [master's thesis]. Stanford, Calif: Stanford University; 1978.

43. Dunkel RH. Survey of attitudes of Arkansas physicians and physical therapists toward the professional capacity of the physical therapist. *Phys Ther* 1974;54(6):584-587.

44. Senters JM. Professionalization in a health occupation: Physical therapy. *Phys Ther* 1972;52(4): 385-392.

45. Website of the American Physical Therapy Association. Accessed Nov 10, 2003. Available at: http://www.apta.org/Education/dpt/dpt_faq#BM6.

46. Swisher LL, Beckstead JW, Bebeau MJ. Factor analysis as a tool for survey analysis using professional role orientation inventory as an example. *Phys Ther* 2004;84:784-799.

47. *Professionalism in physical therapy. Consensus document of the American Physical Therapy Association.* Alexandria, Va: American Physical Therapy Association; 2003.

48. Jette DU, Portney LG. Construct validation of a model for professional behavior in physical therapist students. *Phys Ther* 2003;83:432-443.

49. MacDonald CA, Houghton P, Cox PD, et al. Consensus on physical therapy professional behaviors. *Physiother Canada* 2001;53:212-218, 222.

50. Lopopolo RB. Development of the professional role behaviors survey (PROBES). *Phys Ther* 2001; 81(7):1317-1327.

51. Lopopolo RB. Hospital restructuring and the changing nature of the physical therapist's role. *Phys Ther* 1999;79(2):171-185.

52. Threlkeld AJ, Jensen GM, Royeen CB. The clinical doctorate: A framework for analysis in physical therapist education. *Phys Ther* 1999;79(6):567-581.

53. May WW, Morgan BJ, Lemke JC, et al. Model for ability-based assessment in physical therapy education. *J Phys Ther Educ* 1995;9(1):3-6.

54. Hart E, Pinkston D, Ritchey FJ, et al. Relationship of professional involvement to clinical behaviors of physical therapists. *Phys Ther* 1990;70(13):179-187.

55. Wise D. Oath compilation summary. Unpublished manuscript distributed via electronic mail, 10/28/2003. Used with permission of the author.

56. El-Din, D. Teaching diagnosis. *J Physical Ther Educ* 1995;2:34.

2

The History of a Profession

A society, a profession, without a sense of the past for which it has respect, lacks identity and regard for the future.

Helen Hislop

Hislop H. Tenth Mary McMillan Lecture: The not so-impossible dream. Phys Ther 1975;55:1010-1080.

A generation which ignores history has no past and no future.

Robert Heinlein

Heinlein R. The Notebooks of Lazurus Long. Riverdale, NY: Baen Books, 2004

SHARED HISTORY AS A KEY TO PROFESSIONALIZATION

A look at professional organizations in general provides the foundation for an understanding of the role of the American Physical Therapy Association (APTA) in the development and history of the physical therapy profession. A professional organization fulfills a number of functions for its members and the profession as a whole and establishes a framework for meeting these responsibilities. The following are functions of a professional organization[1]:

- Advancing the economic and social welfare of the practitioners in a profession
- Consolidating practitioners into a single organization
- Providing social and moral support to help members perform their duties
- Reinforcing the strongest members rather than catering to the weakest
- Enabling practitioners to perform their professional duties more easily so as to further benefit patients
- Helping to prepare practitioners for their professional roles and advance their education
- Promoting legal and professional standards of competence
- Developing social and moral ties among members for a community of purpose

The following are the obligations of a professional organization[1]:

- Setting standards for practice and research in the profession
- Helping to ensure the qualification of those recruited into the profession
- Maintaining the profession's traditions

- Anticipating the future of the profession and continually raising the bar of expectations
- Advancing well-founded research and establishing journals for reporting that research
- Justifying the (frequently expanding) scope of the profession
- Developing a consensus so that the organization can speak authoritatively on behalf of the profession, yet at the same time encouraging different viewpoints
- Providing opportunities for communication of members' interests and concerns through democratically elected representatives

Associations provide the social bonds that allow their practitioners to act as a single body. Each association serves as a mediator for the profession in many interactions, including those involving practitioners themselves, the organizations in which they practice, third-party payers, other professional associations, universities, and the government.[1] Few would deny that the APTA has more than met the challenge of serving as a strong professional association for the specialty of physical therapy, and the history of the organization reflects the development of the discipline.

As Terlouw[2] points out, a shared history is one of the strongest bonds of any social group. A group's history is one of the keys to professionalization, because this history is the means by which the group defines itself and determines its mission and goals. To forge a collective identity, therefore, physical therapists (PTs) must build on their shared knowledge of the past. Studying the development of physical therapy as a profession reminds members of their achievements, alerts them to current possibilities, and projects the future of their profession. The history can also help answer these questions[2]:

- What binds the members of the profession into a unified group?
- What professional relationships exist between PTs and other health care specialists? How did these relationships evolve?
- Why were laws enacted to regulate the practice of physical therapy? Do the reasons for enacting these laws still apply?
- What makes the practice of physical therapy different from country to country?
- What new problems does the profession face? What old problems persist?
- What values do PTs consider important?
- How has the perception of the PT's role changed—both within the profession and without?

In general, PTs have an undeveloped historical consciousness of their profession and undervalue its history, in part because professional historians have made few attempts to develop a history of the profession. Terlouw[2] points out that this results in a "collective amnesia" about the specialty. The United States, Australia, Norway, the United Kingdom, and the Netherlands have made the most progress in archiving historical documents about physical therapy.[2]

This chapter provides a synopsis of the history of physical therapy in the United States within a broader social context and explores key events in the creation and development of the APTA, the professional voice of PTs in the United States.

EVOLUTION OF PHYSICAL THERAPY

Social History

Wars, epidemics, accidents, the needs of the physically handicapped, and an increased social demand for integration of people with disabilities into society have all shaped the development of physical therapy as an essential component of health care.[3] Federal legislation and medical advances also have contributed to the evolution of the profession.

Table 2-1 | Important Events in the History of Physical Therapy: 1910-1939

	1910-1919	1920-1929	1930-1939
Major social events	1903: Wright brothers initiate era of flight. 1911: Structure of the atom is discovered. 1912: *Titanic* sinks. 1917: United States enters World War I. 1918: Worldwide influenza epidemic kills millions.	1920: Women win right to vote (Nineteenth Amendment). 1925: Scopes "monkey trial" tests theory of evolution. 1927: First talking movie is produced. 1927: Lindbergh flies nonstop across Atlantic Ocean. 1928: Penicillin is discovered 1929: Stock market crashes.	1932: Atom is split. 1937: National Foundation for Infantile Paralysis is created. 1939: Helicopter is invented.
Health care and other legislation	1906: U.S. Food and Drug Administration (FDA) is created. 1916: Workmen's Compensation Act is passed. 1917: Army's Division of Special Hospitals and Physical Reconstruction is created.	1920: Volstead Act launches Prohibition. 1922: Federal Narcotics Control Board is created.	1930: Veterans Administration is established. 1933: Volstead Act is repealed. 1935: Social Security Act is passed.
Medical milestones	1901: Blood groups are discovered. 1903: Electrocardiogram (EKG) is invented. 1912: Vitamins are introduced.	1923: Nobel Prize is awarded to Banting and Macleod for discovery of insulin. 1927: Iron lung is invented. 1929: Blueprint for modern health insurance is created.	1932: Sulfa drugs are created. 1939: First Blue Shield insurance plan for physician fees is established.

Continued

Table 2-1 | Important Events in the History of Physical Therapy: 1910-1939—cont'd

	1910-1919	1920-1929	1930-1939
Physical therapy landmarks	1913: Pennsylvania becomes first state to license PTs. 1917: Marguerite Sanderson is hired as director of the Reconstruction Aide program. 1918: Fifteen schools for Reconstruction Aides are established.	1921: American Women's Physical Therapeutic Association is formed; Mary McMillan is elected first president. 1921: McMillan publishes first physical therapy text. 1922: First AWPTA convention is held; name is changed to American Physiotherapy Association (APA). 1926: Monthly publication of *Physiotherapy Review* begins. 1927: New York University establishes first 4-year bachelor of science degree program for PTs.	1933: APA asks the American Medical Association (AMA) for assistance with accreditation. 1935: AMA creates the American Registry for PTs who pass a qualifying examination. 1935: APTA *Code of Ethics* is established.

The first decades of the twentieth century were exciting times in the development of physical therapy, with many firsts occurring: Pennsylvania became the first state to license PTs; the first physical therapy textbook and the first journal devoted to physical therapy were published; and the first baccalaureate program for PTs was established (Table 2-1). The creation of the American Women's Physical Therapeutic Association (AWPTA) coincided with passage of the Nineteenth Amendment, which gave women the right to vote. The political action of the suffragettes may have encouraged the small group of "reconstruction aides" to create this new profession for women in the aftermath of World War I, as the United States developed programs to provide care for injured soldiers, workers, and the children devastated by the effects of infantile paralysis, or poliomyelitis (known simply as polio).

The polio epidemics of this era resulted in devastating disability for millions of people worldwide, including President Franklin D. Roosevelt.[4] Although Roosevelt dominated the times from his wheelchair, the general public was not aware of the extent of his functional disability. Only 2 of the 35,000 still photographs of Roosevelt show him seated in a wheelchair, and no newsreels show him being lifted, carried, or pushed in the wheelchair.[4] The extent of the efforts to conceal Roosevelt's limitations demonstrates the challenge faced by physical therapy pioneers; even as they treated thousands of soldiers with severe war-related conditions and innumerable civilians with physical disabilities, these early practitioners worked to gain recognition of their newly emerging profession as an important component of health care.

The years 1940 to 1969 were marked by the passage of legislation supporting the training of allied health personnel, the building of hospitals, and the creation of Medicare and Medicaid (Table 2-2). Soldiers injured in World War II and in Korea and Vietnam required the attention of PTs in the military and in Veterans Administration hospitals. The development of the Salk vaccine in 1952 all but eliminated polio in the United States. However, the demand for PTs did not diminish; rather, it continued to grow. Medicare and Medicaid recipients required rehabilitation services, and with technological advances in cardiac and orthopedic surgery making bed rest as a means of recuperation a thing of the past, the roles of PTs in postsurgical rehabilitation expanded.

In 1956 the American Physiotherapy Association (formerly the AWPTA) changed its name to the American Physical Therapy Association and became more structurally complex through the creation of special interest groups and sections. By moving its home office to Washington, D.C. in the late 60s and expanding its paid staff, the organization positioned itself to take a more active role in the federal political process. As a result of the APTA's efforts, the first nationwide licensure examination was developed, and licensure of PTs in all jurisdictions was mandated. The Physical Therapy Fund, which supports research in the profession, and the first postbaccalaureate degree program for entry level PTs were established. Staffing shortages in the 1960s resulted in creation of the physical therapist assistant (PTA) position and an influx of PTs from other countries.

Legislation to control health care costs and to increase accountability for services dominated the final decades of the twentieth century (Table 2-3). Even as new laws ensured the rights of children and adults with disabilities, funding for health care services was tightened by legislation that limited hospital construction and expansion, shifted the reimbursement process to prospective payments for hospital stays, and reduced health care spending through the new managed care models. Rising concerns about the impact of chronic conditions on health care costs paralleled medical advances in preventing disease and prolonging life, which generated new bioethical issues.

Text continued on p. 32

Table 2-2 | **Important Events in the History of Physical Therapy: 1940-1969**

	1940-1949	1950-1959	1960-1969
Major social events	1941: Pearl Harbor is attacked; United States enters World War II. 1944: President Roosevelt launches the New Deal. 1945: First computer is built. 1948: Israel is founded. 1949: China becomes a Communist nation.	1950: Korean War begins. 1950: First credit card is issued. 1951: Atom bomb is created. 1955: American Federation of Labor (AFL) and Congress of Industrial Organizations (CIO) merge; organized labor's goals include bargaining for health insurance benefits. 1957: Sputnik is launched. 1959: Castro becomes dictator of Cuba.	1961: Soviets launch first manned space flight. 1961: Berlin wall is built. 1963: President Kennedy is assassinated. 1963: Betty Friedan's *Feminine Mystique* is published. 1965: U.S. troops are sent to Vietnam. 1967: First Super Bowl game is played. 1968: Martin Luther King, Jr. and Robert Kennedy are assassinated. 1969: Neil Armstrong is first person to land on the moon. 1969: Yassar Arafat becomes leader of the Palestine Liberation Organization.
Health care and other legislation	1946: Hill-Burton Act provides funds for the creation and building of hospitals.	1953: Allied Health Professional Training Act is passed.	1964: Civil Rights Act is passed, establishing the Equal Employment Opportunity Commission. 1965: Social Security amendments create Medicare (Title XVIII) and Medicaid (Title XIX).
Medical milestones	1946: Physical medicine physicians become known as *physiatrists*. 1948: Cortisone is first used for arthritis.	1950: First school of allied health is created. 1950: First organ transplant is performed. 1951: Joint Commission on Accreditation of Hospitals is created.	1960: Birth control pill is developed. 1962: FDA amendments require premarket approval of drugs.

	1952: Salk vaccine is developed.	1951: World Congress of Physical Therapy is created.	1960: First graduate program in physical therapy is established at Case Western Reserve University.
	1952: First open heart surgery is performed.	1953: Section on Private Practice is formed.	1965: APTA Section on Research is formed.
	1953: Deoxyribonucleic acid (DNA) is discovered.	1954: Professional Examination Services competency examination is developed.	1966: PTs serve in Vietnam on the front lines.
	1954: Tobacco is linked to incidence of cancer.	1956: APA becomes the American Physical Therapy Association (APTA).	1966: Position of PTA is created in response to staffing shortages; recruitment and immigration of PTs from other countries increases.
	1957: Informed consent is incorporated into medical care.	1957: Physical Therapy Fund is formed to further research.	
	1958: Total hip arthroplasty is developed.		
Physical therapy landmarks	1941: First special interest groups meet; first continuing education programs are held.		
	1944: APA House of Delegates is created; organization moves to first national office in New York, N.Y.		

Table 2-3 | **Focus of Ethics Literature in Physical Therapy: 1970-1999**

	1970-1979	1980-1989	1990-1999
Major social events	1970: Computer floppy disk is introduced. 1971: Videocassette recorder (VCR) is invented. 1971: Watergate scandal occurs. 1971: United States ends Vietnam War. 1973: Abortion is legalized. 1974: President Nixon resigns. 1975: Microsoft is founded. 1979: Iran takes American hostages.	1980: Cable News Network (CNN) is created. 1981: First woman is appointed to the U.S. Supreme Court. 1983: "Star Wars" defense plan is launched. 1985: Hole in the ozone layer is discovered. 1985: Soviets proclaim *perestroika* and *glasnost.* 1986: Mir space station is launched. 1988: Pan American airliner explodes over Lockerbie, Scotland. 1989: *Exxon Valdez* oil spill occurs.	1991: South Africa ends apartheid. 1992: Cold War ends. 1993: Internet grows exponentially. 1993: European Union is formed. 1995: Federal building in Oklahoma City is bombed. 1997: First sheep is cloned. 1999: Y2K computer scare arises.
Health care and other legislation	1973: Health Maintenance Organization Act is passed. 1973: Section 504 of the Rehabilitation Act prohibits discrimination based on disability in federal programs. 1974: National Health Planning and Resources Development Act requires Certificate of Needs for federal funds. 1975: Individuals with Disabilities Education Act (IDEA) is passed.	1982: Tax Equity and Fiscal Responsibility Act creates diagnostic related groups. 1984: Peer review organizations are organized. 1989: Agency for Healthcare Research and Quality is created. 1989: Omnibus Budget Reconciliation Act is passed.	1990: Americans with Disabilities Act is passed. 1990: Patient Self-Determination Act is passed. 1990: National Center for Rehabilitation Research is created. 1996: HIPAA is enacted. 1997: Balanced Budget Act is passed (includes PACE program). 1999: Immigration and Naturalization Service rules affect foreign-trained physical therapists and other health care workers.

Medical milestones

1972: First computed axial tomography (CAT) scan is performed.
1978: First test tube baby is born.

1981: Acquired immunodeficiency syndrome (AIDS) is identified.
1987: Joint Commission on Accreditation of Hospitals becomes the Joint Commission on Accreditation of Healthcare Organizations.

1990: Genome project begins.
1996: "Mad cow" disease devastates herds in Britain.

Physical therapy landmarks

1973 Affiliate membership in APTA for PTA is created.
1973: New York University establishes first doctoral program in physical therapy.
1974: First PT school is established in a historically black university (Howard University).
1976: First combined sections meeting is held.
1976: PT Registry is disbanded.

1981: First Foundation for Physical Therapy research grants are awarded.
1983: Commission on Accreditation for Physical Therapy Education becomes sole accrediting body for PT education.
1985: Board certification of specialists in PT is established.
1988: APTA Minority Affairs department is created.
1988: Tri-alliance (physical therapy, occupational therapy, and speech language pathology) is established.

1993: First DPT degree program is established at Creighton University.
1995: *Guide to Physical Therapist Practice* is published.
1998: APTA membership is reorganized into the American College of Physical Therapists and the National Assembly of Physical Therapist Assistants.

During this time the APTA became solely responsible for the accreditation of PT educational programs, developed specialty sections and specialty certification, and defined itself through the *Guide to Physical Therapist Practice*, published in 1997.[5] The first doctoral program in physical therapy was created, the Foundation for Physical Therapy awarded its first research grants, and the first specialists in physical therapy were certified. The APTA subcategorized its members into the American College of Physical Therapists and the National Assembly of Physical Therapist Assistants.

Pioneers of Physical Therapy

Physical therapy could not have evolved into the profession it is today without the vision of its pioneers. The history of physical therapy in the United States begins with Mary McMillan, who founded the American Women's Physiotherapy Association and was elected its first president in 1921. Although American born, McMillan lived in Europe in her early years. She completed studies at Liverpool University and did graduate work in physical culture and corrective exercises, which included Swedish gymnastics and the dynamics of scoliosis. She then worked in hospitals in England, where she treated victims of industrial accidents, children with polio and developmental deformities, and the war wounded, until she returned to the United States in 1915. McMillan became director of massage and medical gymnastics at the Children's Hospital in Portland, Maine.[6]

Her interest in body movement may have been influenced by events in England at that time. In 1894 four nurses had founded the Society of Trained Masseuses, which in 1920 merged with the Institute of Massage and Remedial Gymnastics (which became the Chartered Society of Physiotherapists in 1944[7]). It is interesting that the founders of physiotherapy in England were nurses, whereas in the United States, early recruits into what would become the profession of physical therapy were primarily women with physical education degrees.

In addition to McMillan, a number of others proved influential in the emergence of the discipline of physical therapy during the first decades of the twentieth century. These included Dr. Frank Granger, a physician who taught physical therapeutics at Harvard's Graduate School of Medicine and applied the techniques in his neurology practice, as well as Dr. Elliott Brackett and Dr. Joel Goldthwait, chief surgeons in the Army's Orthopedic Military Corps.[8] In 1917, as World War I raged, the surgeon general of the U.S. Army, Major General William Gorgas, anticipated the need for a formal reconstruction program for injured soldiers, such as had already been established in some European countries. He established the Army's Division of Special Hospitals and Physical Reconstruction, which was charged with the development of educational programs to prepare "reconstruction aides." Granger, Brackett, and Goldthwait were recruited to create emergency training programs for reconstruction aides in physical therapy and in occupational therapy.[8] Many of the interventions used by future PTs are grounded in the work of these physicians.

Marguerite Sanderson, a graduate of the Boston Normal School of Gymnastics who had worked with Dr. Goldthwait, was sent to Walter Reed General Hospital in Washington, D.C., to organize units of the Reconstruction Aide Corps, which were to be sent to overseas hospitals. McMillan was appointed a reconstruction aide, and she arrived at Walter Reed General Hospital as Sanderson headed to Europe to oversee her trainees. The armistice ending the war in 1918 soon followed.[8]

Over the next two years, McMillan developed and served as an instructor for the most far-reaching emergency training program for reconstruction aides, at Reed

College in Portland, Oregon. She also wrote *Massage and Therapeutic Exercise*,[9] the first physical therapy textbook. Subsequently, she became the superintendent of physical therapy reconstruction aides in the U.S. surgeon general's office, and six more emergency training centers for reconstruction aides were established to meet the expected onslaught of war wounded. Upon their return to the United States, 86,000 soldiers received care from the reconstruction aides.[6] In 1920, with the need for military reconstruction aides dwindling, McMillan accepted a position with Dr. Brackett in his practice and later helped develop graduate programs for PTs at Harvard with Dr. Granger.[8]

As the reconstruction aides began to scatter into civilian positions, McMillan proposed the establishment of a national association to preserve the role of PTs, who had proved their value in the new rehabilitation component of health care. She contacted 800 potential members, inviting them to form the AWPTA; the annual fee would be $2. McMillan received 120 replies, and an organizational meeting was held on January 15, 1921, in New York. Primarily driven by their need for recognition of the duties they now performed through the public health service, in the newly created veterans' hospitals, and in hospitals for crippled children, the members of the AWPTA adopted a constitution, established bylaws, and elected McMillan their first president.[8]

Any individual whose physical therapy training and experience was comparable to or exceeded that of the reconstruction aides was invited to join, and 274 members from 32 states were added in the first year.[8] The first issue of the *Physical Therapy Review*, the AWPTA journal, soon appeared, with a call for the setting of standards in the education of PTs.[8]

The AWPTA's first annual conference, in 1922, included a business meeting, educational programs, and time for socializing (much as do APTA conferences today). The organization's name was officially changed to the American Physiotherapy Association (APA) at this meeting.[8]

What to call themselves in the world of work became a major issue for APA members during the 1920s. The terms *physiotherapist, physiotherapeutist, physical therapist*, and *physical therapy technician* all were suggested. However, this seemingly simple decision was complicated by the concurrent emergence of a small group of physicians who used electrotherapeutics and physical modalities in their treatments and who were attempting to distinguish themselves from other medical specialties. This group laid claim to the term *physiotherapist*, and their physician organization, the American Congress of Physical Therapy, began a campaign to ensure that only physicians could use the term *physical therapist*. The organization argued that the public was accustomed to thinking that any title ending in "-ist" was associated with a physician, such as neurologist or radiologist; therefore use of the term *physical therapist* by those who were not physicians would be misleading the public. The physicians' organization recommended that the APA use the term *physiotherapy technician*. The APA held its ground, and in 1930 it incorporated in Illinois, ensuring its legal title (changed to APTA in 1956). Nevertheless, many practitioners referred to themselves as "physical therapy technicians" to appease physicians.[6] Physicians now use the term *physiatrists* for specialists in physical medicine and rehabilitation.

As a result of these early efforts, the APTA's current membership exceeds 60,000, and the organization is a powerful force in addressing the contemporary issues of the profession (see Chapter 3). Box 2-1 presents a comparison of the preamble to the AWPTA's constitution, written in 1921, with the annual goals of the APTA established in 2004. The comparison shows how far the profession has come.

Box 2-1   Goals of Physical Therapy Professional Organizations: Then and Now

American Women's Physical Therapeutic Association (1921)

AWPTA Constitution: Article II Objects, Section 1

The purpose of this association shall be to establish and maintain a professional and scientific standard for those engaged in the profession of physical therapeutics; to increase efficiency among its members by encouraging them in advanced study; to disseminate information by the distribution of medical literature and articles of professional interest; to assist in securing positions for its members; to make available efficiently trained women to the medical profession; and to sustain social fellowship and intercourse upon grounds of mutual interest.

Priority Goals of the American Physical Therapy Association (APTA) (2004)

Goal I: PTs are universally recognized and promoted as the practitioners of choice for persons with conditions that affect movement, function, health, and wellness.

Goal II: Academic and clinical education prepares doctors of physical therapy who are autonomous practitioners.

Goal III: PTs are autonomous practitioners to whom patients/clients have unrestricted direct access as an entry point into the health care delivery system and who are paid for all elements of patient/client management in all practice environments.

Goal IV: Research advances the science of physical therapy and furthers the evidence-based practice of the PT.

Goal V: PTs and PTAs are committed to meeting the health needs of patients/clients and society through ethical behavior, continued competence, and advocacy for the profession.

Goal VI: Communication throughout the Association enhances participation and responsiveness to members and instills the value of belonging to the APTA.

Goal VII: APTA standards, policies, positions, guidelines and the *Guide to Physical Therapist Practice, Normative Model of Physical Therapist Education and Evaluative Criteria,* and the *Normative Model of Physical Therapist Assistant Education and Evaluative Criteria* are recognized and used as the foundation for physical therapist practice, research, and education environments.

These goals are based upon the APTA Vision Statement for Physical Therapy 2020 (Vision 2020) developed by the Association in 2000. The goals encompass the Association's major priorities as it moves toward realization of the ideals set forth in Vision 2020. The Board is committed to these goals as the foundation from which to lead the Association. The Association's awareness of cultural diversity, its commitment to expanding minority representation and participation in physical therapy, and its commitment to equal opportunity for all members suffuse these goals. These goals are not ranked and do not represent any priority order.

Physical Therapy Today

The APTA has performed well in fulfilling the functions of a professional organization and in meeting its obligations to its members. Through its political action and lobbying efforts, it has protected the economic and social welfare of its members, particularly in the area of health care financing legislation. The influence of the APTA on licensure requirements and on ethical, educational, and research standards directly affects the performance of each individual practitioner's professional duties.

The APTA continues to meet its obligations as a professional organization by successfully anticipating the future; by raising practice expectations for PTs and PTAs through consistent updating of the standards of practice, professional code of ethics, and guides for professional conduct; through development of the physical therapy research agenda (and by providing funds for this research); and by crafting *Physical Therapy* into a respected, peer-reviewed journal.

Through its activities, and particularly with the rise of electronic media, the APTA has provided numerous means of communication for its members. On topics ranging from broad professional questions to specific daily practice and educational issues, members share information and guide the association's decisions. Conferences on contemporary issues and the presentation of research studies and innovative ideas at annual APTA meetings also provide forums for open discussion of professional issues. The APTA also offers continuing education courses at seminars and on-line.

Another APTA strength has been the management of "turf wars," which have arisen as the scope of the PT profession has expanded over the years and as other professions have attempted breeches of the physical therapy boundaries of practice. Since the early days, when physicians were reluctant to legitimize the role of PTs in health care, the APTA has monitored the activities of professional organizations for chiropractors, kinesiotherapists, athletic trainers, exercise physiologists, and occupational therapists, as these associations seek to meet their obligations to their members to expand the scope of their professions.

DEVELOPMENT OF VALUES

Ethical Issues

Examining the ethical challenges that a profession addresses over time is integral to understanding its history. In her address for the 2000 Mary McMillan Lecture, Ruth Purtilo[10] used the metaphor "seeds of care and accountability" adapting to the "social landscape" to describe the evolution of physical therapy over three identity periods: self-identity, patient-focused identity, and societal identity. During the period of self-identity (beginning with the first code of ethics, published in 1935 by the APA), ethical issues arose primarily around interactions with other professionals, not an unexpected development as the first PTs sought to clarify their relationships with physicians and occupational therapists as they moved into civilian roles. Ethical issues during the period of patient-focused identity (beginning about 1950) centered primarily on the professional relationship with patients and on patients' rights, reflecting the broader civil rights issues of the times and the inclusion of informed consent as a routine component of medical care. The third, and current, identity period encompasses the concerns of the previous two. PTs must now partner with institutions and the community so that their self-identity and patients' interests are "nested in societal accountability" (Figure 2-1).

Using Purtilo's three periods, Swisher[11] evaluated peer-reviewed articles on ethics knowledge from 1970 to 2000 (Table 2-4). She concluded that the literature did in fact conform to these general time periods. The current trend toward partnerships may be partly the result of legislation that empowered patients (e.g., the Patient Self-Determination and the Americans with Disabilities Acts), created health maintenance organizations, and demanded greater fiscal responsibility from health care organizations. A striking finding of this study was the relative dearth of ethics publications over the years (only 90 peer-reviewed ethics articles appeared in major health databases), which suggests the need for further exploration of this aspect of the development of the profession.

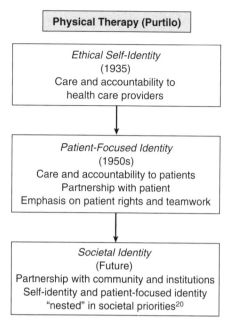

Figure 2-1. Purtilo's three periods of ethics in physical therapy. (*Modified from Swisher LL. A retrospective analysis of ethics knowledge in physical therapy (1970-2000). Phys Ther 2002; 82:692-706.*)

Professional Recognition

A review of the accomplishments that a profession chooses to recognize can also provide insight into the evolution of a profession's values. The annual Mary McMillan Lecture Award, presented since 1964, highlights the achievements that the physical therapy profession has deemed most important.

Mary McMillan, the early guiding spirit of the physical therapy profession, led the way to higher standards in treatment and started PTs on the road toward greater professional service to their patients. The APTA created the Mary McMillan Lecture Award in her honor after her death in 1959. The award honors members of the APTA who have made a distinguished contribution to the profession in more than one of the areas of administration, education, patient care, and research. Candidates are judged on the depth, scope, duration, and quality of their contributions and their wide-reaching effects on the image of the profession. Recipients share their achievements and ideas with members in an address presented at the APTA's annual conference, which is then published in the November issue of *Physical Therapy* each year (Table 2-5).

The topics chosen by those honored can be said to reflect the issues the profession has identified as significant to its image and the evolving role of the PT in practice, research, and education. The predominant theme in the lectures of the 1990s was the scholarly role of PTs and the need for research and a scientific basis for practice. The education and role of faculty, accountability, and decision making by PTs are other topics that have been addressed. These themes reflect the enduring values of the small group of women who founded the profession almost a hundred years ago.

Table 2-4 | **Descriptive Model of the Evolution of Ethics Positions in Physical Therapy**

Elements	1970-1979	1980-1989	1990-2000
Approach	Philosophical* Professional/historical	Philosophical Application of	Philosophical and social scientific (equal numbers)
Issues/topics	Historical context Physical therapist as ethical decision maker Teaching of ethics Research and informed consent	principles to physical therapy problems Justice in resource allocation Informed consent Ethical responsibility in autonomous practice	Managed care and scarce resources Discrimination and prejudice Relationship between physical therapist and patient/client Theoretical models of physical therapy that embrace ethics
Role of the physical therapist*	Patient/client management Critical inquiry Administrator Educator	Patient/client management Critical inquiry	Patient/client management Educator Administrator Critical inquiry
Identity (Purtilo[10])	Self-identity and patient-focused identity	Patient-focused identity	Patient-focused identity (growing societal identity)
Recurrent themes	Need to identify ethical issues encountered by physical therapists Close relationship between clinical and ethical decision making Changing relationship with patient (from hierarchical to mutual models)		

Modified from Swisher LL. A retrospective analysis of ethics knowledge in physical therapy (1970-2000). Phys Ther 2002;82:692-706.
*Patterns of focus are listed in descending order of frequency.

THE WORLD CONFEDERATION FOR PHYSICAL THERAPY

The evolution of physical therapy in other countries provides a broader perspective on the development of the profession as a whole. The World Confederation for Physical Therapy (WCPT), with 11 founding members (Australia, Canada, Denmark, Finland, Great Britain, New Zealand, Norway, South Africa, Sweden, the United States, and West Germany), held its first session in 1951.[4] Currently the WCPT has 82 member organizations, which represent more than 225,000 PTs worldwide.[6] WCPT purposes are as follows[12]:
- Representing physical therapy and PTs internationally
- Collaborating with national and other international organizations
- Encouraging high standards of physical therapy research, education, and practice
- Supporting communication and the exchange of information among regions and member organizations

The challenges a professional association faces in carrying out its functions and obligations are significantly compounded when the task requires a global effort involving numerous member associations. Looking out for the social and economic

Text continued on p. 43

Table 2-5 | **APTA Mary McMillan Lectures and Their Professional Messages***

Year	Lecturer	Title	Professional Messages
1964	Mildred O. Elson	"The Legacy of Mary McMillan"	Discussed the qualities of Mary McMillan and the beginnings of the profession.
1965	Catherine Worthingham	"Complementary Functions and Responsibilities in an Emerging Profession"	Noted that academic and clinical physical therapists were preparing for a changing environment, complementing each others' work and presenting a united front as a true profession.
1966	Ruby Decker	"A Hard Look"	Reaffirmed the roles of the physical therapist (PT) as clinician, researcher, administrator, consultant, and educator who supervises others, as well as those of student, professional (ethics/legal), and citizen involved in community affairs. Called for PTs to assume management of PT departments and to control accreditation and the preparation of support personnel.
1967	Emma E. Vogel	"The History of Physical Therapists: The United States Army"	Presented a history of PTs in the army through the Vietnam War.
1968	Helen L. Kaiser	"Today's Tomorrow"	Examined PTs' relationship to other professionals with regard to allied health and physical medicine and rehabilitation issues.
1969	Margaret S. Rood	"Stereotyped or Integrated Response"	Not published.
1971	Lucy Blair	"Past Experiences Project Future Responsibilities"	Noted that, 50 years after the profession was created to establish the role of physical therapy in health care, PTs' commitment to high standards of excellence was critical.
1972	Margaret Knott	"In the Groove"	Discussed the importance of international relations in physical therapy and global participation in the community of physical therapy; also argued for proprioceptive neuromuscular facilitation.
1973	Lucille Daniels	"Tomorrow Now: The Master's Degree for Physical Therapy Education"	Proposed that master's degree serve as the entry-level degree for PTs.

Year	Name	Title	Description
1975	Helen J. Hislop	"The Not-So-Impossible Dream"	Examined the importance of the scientific foundation of physical therapy, which was suggested to be pathokinesiology, the need for specialization in physical therapy, and identification of the PT's unique role in health care, affecting individuals from the cellular to the family level.
1976	Eleanor J. Carlin	"The Revolutionary Spirit"	Pointed out the need to persuade patients of the value of PTs (i.e., consumer identification of physical therapy).
1977	Mary Clyde Singleton	"Do We Dare to Remember?"	Discussed the art of physical therapy, specifically the balance of its scientific and humanistic aspects.
1978	Margaret L. Moore	"Building Winning Teams"	Emphasized the importance of leadership in clinical and academic physical therapy and the interrelationship of the two approaches.
1979	Helen Blood	"Account Ability"	Presented a model of societal influences on health care functions and the incurred obligations of PTs.
1980	Florence P. Kendall	"This I Believe"	Discussed procedures for bylaws, the need to test the PT's knowledge of state law, and the potential of individuals to make a difference.
1981	Susanne P. Hirt	"Progress Is a Relay Race"	Addressed specialization and the postbaccalaureate degree.
1982	Dorothy E. Voss	"Everything Is There Before You Discover It"	Discussed proprioceptive neuromuscular facilitation and rededication to patient care.
1983	Nancy T. Watts	"The Privilege of Choice"	Examined decision making with patients and in PT education, as well as the scope of PT practice.
1984	Eugene Michaels	"Nineteenth Mary McMillan Lecture"	Pointed out the importance of argument, philosophy, ideology, and rhetoric in the development of physical therapy.
1985	Geneva R. Johnson	"Great Expectations: A Force in Growth and Change"	Stated predictions for 2005 (i.e., schools of physical therapy outside of academic institutions, PTs as service contractors rather than employees, research aspects, clearly delineated roles of the physical therapist assistant).
1986	Dorothy Pinkston	"Twenty-First Mary McMillan Lecture"	Explained the high tangible and intangible costs of growth of the APTA and in PT education.

Continued

Table 2-5 | **APTA Mary McMillan Lectures and Their Professional Messages***—cont'd

Year	Lecturer	Title	Professional Messages
1987	Charles M. Magistro	"Twenty-Second Mary McMillan Lecture"	Discussed private practice physical therapy and challenges regarding reimbursement.
1989	Ruth Wood	"Footprints"	Discussed independent practice and putting patients first, as well as diagnosis and compliance with ethical standards in a caring, touching profession.
1990	L. Don Lehmkuhl	"Camelot Revisited: Legacy of the Physical Therapy Education Program at Case Western Reserve University"	Examined the role of PT as researcher and the role of Case Western Reserve University in development of the profession.
1991	Robert C. Bartlett	"In Our Hands"	Explored sociopolitical influences on the profession, noting the need to better define the uniqueness of physical therapy.
1992	Marylou R. Barnes	"The Twenty-Sixth Mary McMillan Lecture"	Discussed challenges to the scholarly role of the physical therapy faculty and the need for creativity in clinical education.
1993	Gary L. Soderberg	"On Passing From Ignorance to Knowledge"	Examined scholarship in the academic and clinical settings and the need for clinical research.
1996	Bella J. May	"On Decision Making"	Presented a model of decision making for clinicians and discussed the important decisions made by the American Physical Therapy Association (APTA).
1998	Shirley A. Sahrmann	"Moving Precisely? Or Taking the Path of Least Resistance?"	Proposed establishing movement as a physiological system; also noted the need for a clear clinical science in physical therapy and for acceptance of physical therapy as a true academic unit in universities.
1999	Suzann K. Campbell	"PT 2000: Nurturing the Profession"	Examined the need for research to build the future in Research I academic institutions; the need to improve coordination, communication, and documentation; and the importance of mentoring in the APTA.

2000	Ruth B. Purtilo	"A Time to Harvest, a Time to Sow: Ethics for a Shifting Landscape"	Explored the "seasons" of professional ethics in physical therapy, including the movement from self-identity to patient focus and societal identity and the need for deeper respect for all individuals and for cultural diversity in physical therapy.
2001	Jules M. Rothstein	"Journeys Beyond the Horizon"	Explained that the scientific, accountability, and humanistic principles of the physical therapy profession make it unique and essential; also explored the accountability of the profession's leadership.
2002	Steven L. Wolf	"'Look Forward, Walk Tall'": Exploring Our 'What If' Questions"	Redefined professionalism as essential and esoteric; also discussed the potential impact of genetics on physical therapy. In addition, challenged professionals to ask the *whats* and *whys* of what is taught in physical therapy education, to link interventions to changes in patient behavior, and to include research and education within APTA sections rather than treat them as separate sections.
2003	Pamela W. Duncan	"One Grip a Little Stronger"	Examined the need for purpose, passion, and perseverance to achieve the vision of the profession, as well as the importance of networking beyond the profession; also called for a shift in focus, to promoting the outcomes of physical therapy rather than the therapists themselves.
2004	Marilyn Moffat	"Braving New Worlds: To Conquer, to Endure"	Presented technological advances in medicine and physical therapy that impact the role of PT. Suggested that regardless of this progress, there will always be a need for physical therapy, particularly the unique skill in therapeutic exercise.

APTA, *American Physical Therapy Association.*

The Mary McMillan Lecture is published in the November issue of Physical Therapy *each year that it is presented. The McMillan Award is not presented every year.*

Table 2-6 | **Selected Member Associations of the World Confederation for Physical Therapy**

Country/Association	Association Founded	Members	Purpose	Web Site
Finland (Finnish Association of Physiotherapists)	1943	8200	Promotes physiotherapy in Finnish society and ensures that physiotherapists are capable of providing high-quality physiotherapy services. Actively follows developments in Finnish society, provides statements, takes stands on issues, presents proposals, and introduces initiatives.	http://www.fysioterapia.net/english/association.html
Ireland (Irish Society of Chartered Physiotherapists)	1983	1300	Represents chartered physiotherapists in Ireland and supports them in the achievement of the highest standards of professional practice. The organization is committed to provision of a health service that is accessible, effective, and humanitarian.	http://www.iscp.ie/content/soc.html
Philippines (Philippine Physical Therapy Association)	1964	1224	Supports the professional development of physical therapists practicing in the Philippines by providing continuing education activities, facilitating access to international publications, and disseminating and using research and development pertinent to physical therapy practice in the Philippines.	http://www.angelfire.com/home/ppta/m&v.htm
Taiwan (Physical Therapy Association of the Republic of China)	1975	2500	Maintains high standards of practice and provides mechanisms for sharing information and experience in the profession, nationwide and internationally.	http://www.ptaroc.org.tw/eng/en1.htm

welfare of member associations around the globe and consolidating their power seems a daunting undertaking, particularly when each member association is at a different stage of development. However, the idea of one association representing all PTs is compelling. Table 2-6 presents information on some of the WCPT's member countries. Whether the course of development for these newer associations follows the historical pattern of older organizations remains to be seen.

FURTHER THOUGHTS

As Marilyn Moffat[13] stated in her presidential address on the 75th anniversary of the APTA, it is fitting to look back and take pride in the history of physical therapy. The destiny of the profession is shaped not only by the force, fervor, and dedication of physical therapy's pioneers but also by the dedicated people who continue to devote themselves to the profession.[13]

Because, like other professionals, PTs often underrate and undervalue the importance of history to their development, the potential for history to provide answers to professional questions remains generally unrealized. The importance of the social role of professional organizations is often dismissed, as reflected in the small percentage of professionals who support them. Merton[1] reminds practitioners who are not members of their professional organizations that they typically receive an unearned increment in moral and economic gain from the work of those organizations. He does not find it inappropriate to call practitioners who remain outside an association "freeloaders" because they do not pay their way either in dues or in kind. He likens them to people who avoid paying taxes yet benefit from the taxes of those who do pay.

QUESTIONS FOR REFLECTION

1. What do you think the current status of physical therapy would be if Mary McMillan hadn't brought former reconstruction aides together to form the AWPTA?
2. What historical events do you think were keys to the activities of the APTA (and its predecessors) in the twentieth century?
3. What do the McMillan lectures and the course of the ethical development of the profession add to our understanding of the history of physical therapy?
4. What are the four key functions of the WCPT?
5. Do you expect the evolution of physical therapy as a profession in other countries to follow the same developmental pattern as that of the APTA? Why or why not?
6. List the most important lessons PTs should learn from the past.

References

1. Merton RK. *Social research and the practicing professions.* Cambridge, Mass: Abt Books; 1982.
2. Terlouw TJA. How can we treat collective amnesia? *Physiotherapy* 2000;86:257-261.
3. Teager DPG. The Molly Levy Eponymous Lecture: The changing profession: An international perspective. *S Afr J Physiother* 1998;54:4-8.
4. Gallagher HG. *FDR's splendid deception.* Arlington, Va: Vandamere Press; 1985.
5. American Physical Therapy Association. Guide to physical therapist practice. *Phys Ther* 1997;77: 1160-1634.

6. Murphy W. *Healing the generations: A history of physical therapy and the American Physical Therapy Association.* Alexandria, Va: American Physical Therapy Association; 1995.

7. Chartered Society of Physiotherapists. *History of the Chartered Society of Physiotherapist.* Retrieved November 13, 2003, at http://www.csp.org.uk/thecsp/about/history.cfm

8. American Physical Therapy Association. The beginning of "modern physiotherapy." *Phys Ther* 1976;56:3-9.

9. McMillan M. *Massage and therapeutic exercise.* Philadelphia: WB Saunders, 1921.

10. Purtilo RB. Thirty-first Mary McMillan Lecture: A time to harvest, a time to sow: Ethics for a shifting landscape. *Phys Ther* 2000;80:1112-1119.

11. Swisher LL. A retrospective analysis of ethics knowledge in physical therapy (1970-2000). *Phys Ther* 2002;82:692-706.

12. World Confederation for Physical Therapy. *Welcome to the World Confederation for Physical Therapy.* Retrieved November 11, 2003, at http://www.wcpt.org

13. Moffat M. 1996 APTA presidential address: Three quarters of a century of healing the generations. *Phys Ther* 1996;76:1242-1252.

Contemporary Practice Issues

We physical therapists are so very capable of imagining new solutions, creating new hope for our patients and clients, and more than braving them, conquering our new worlds.

Marilyn Moffat

Moffat M. Thirty-Fifth Mary McMillan Lecture: Braving new worlds: To conquer, to endure. Phys Ther 2004; 84:1056-1086.

A VISION FOR THE FUTURE

The American Physical Therapy Association (APTA) is the professional voice of physical therapists (PTs) and physical therapist assistants (PTAs) in the United States. The organization has stated its vision for the future as follows[1]:

> Physical therapy, by 2020, will be provided by physical therapists who are doctors of physical therapy and who may be board-certified specialists. Consumers will have direct access to physical therapists in all environments for patient/client management, prevention, and wellness services. Physical therapists will be practitioners of choice in clients' health networks and will hold all privileges of autonomous practice. Physical therapists may be assisted by physical therapist assistants who are educated and licensed to provide physical therapist–directed and –supervised components of interventions.
>
> Guided by integrity, lifelong learning, and a commitment to comprehensive and accessible health programs for all people, physical therapists and physical therapist assistants will render evidence-based service throughout the continuum of care and improve quality of life for society. They will provide culturally sensitive care distinguished by trust, respect, and an appreciation for individual differences.
>
> While fully availing themselves of new technologies, as well as basic and clinical research, physical therapists will continue to provide direct care. They will maintain active responsibility for the growth of the physical therapy profession and the health of the people it serves.

This chapter addresses practice issues raised in the first paragraph of the vision statement, specifically those related to the doctorate of physical therapy (DPT) degree, board certification of specialists, direct access by the public to physical therapy care, and the role of the PTA. The political work of the APTA, which is directed toward making this vision a reality, is also discussed. The issues are explored from two perspectives: the broader one of the profession and the more focused one of individual PTs and their day-to-day practice.

THE DOCTORATE IN PHYSICAL THERAPY

Perspective of the Profession

In 1999, to encourage dialog about the need for the doctor of physical therapy (DPT) degree in the profession, Threlkeld, Jensen, and Royeen,[2] two faculty members and the dean of research at Creighton University, where the first DPT program was started, attempted to determine the influences of the DPT in physical therapy education and the need for the degree program. They published their analysis in the professional journal *Physical Therapy*, arguing that the DPT provides PTs with a clear professional identity consistent with that of other health care professionals (e.g., podiatrists, pharmacists, psychologists, and chiropractors). They further contended that the image of the PT should be consistent with the public's expectations of a professional (i.e., competence, trust, and autonomy of decision making) and that the doctoral degree recognizes and enhances such an image.

The authors also argued that the needs of health care consumers determine not only the demand or need for physical therapy services but also the social status of physical therapy as a profession. They predicted that the following societal trends would necessitate more advanced treatment of patients by PTs, which in turn would require preparation at the doctoral level[2]:

- An ever-increasing number of patients from minority backgrounds
- The use of demographic and epidemiological data to develop physical therapy practice models that would address the changing health care environments in rural and urban areas
- A growing obligation to society to incorporate into clinical practice knowledge gained from both the foundational and the applied sciences
- An expanding understanding of the importance of health beliefs, behaviors, and status in the larger context of health care

Because of these expectations and predicted changes in clinical practice, the authors concluded that PTs require a rigorous and far-reaching education, not merely job training, to prepare them for the future.

Noting a predicted oversupply of those with the doctoral degree by 2005, the authors acknowledged that the market for those with the DPT appeared to be shrinking as a result of changes in the health care system. However, they presented these market changes as an opportunity for PTs to identify new practice opportunities and challenges. Touching on the shrinking pool of applicants to physical therapy programs, the authors raised the possibility that federal loans specific for physical therapy students, as well as other external funding, might become available if doctoral-level programs were in place.[2]

Finally, they argued that adoption of the professional doctoral degree would be advantageous in presenting the professional obligations and responsibilities of PTs in state licensure debates concerning autonomous professional practice. They proposed that DPT programs be located in universities that had at least a doctoral university II rating (or a broad spectrum of professional education) to provide a scholarly and professional context, as well as role models for students.[2] They suggested that the curricula for these DPT programs prepare students for the unpredictable future of clinical practice, which they saw as one in which PTs will be (1) more directly involved in the processes of evaluation, diagnosis, and patient management; (2) delegating and supervising treatment; (3) writing clinical case reports; (4) documenting the use of outcome data; (5) educating patients, families, students, and peers, as well as individuals and agencies not directly involved with the physical therapy profession; and (6) confronting ethical and financial dilemmas imposed by shrinking health care financing.

Responses to these proposals, published in *Physical Therapy* as "Letters to the Editor," covered a range of positions[3]:

- The DPT is the next logical step in the evolution of physical therapy as a profession.
- Little difference in substance exists between the master's and doctoral entry level degrees.
- Given the surplus of PTs, the DPT may be a solution to raising expectations of entry-level PTs to decrease the number entering the profession.
- Before the profession can commit to the DPT as the degree required by society, data need to be collected on the academic environment, program and graduate geographic saturation, and short-term and long-term student outcomes.
- The DPT is an effort to buy the respect of the public and third-party payers with a credential.
- The identified needs regarding management, leadership, and business skills are not actually incorporated into DPT curricula.
- The DPT is needed to meet the demands of the clinical setting and to improve the PT's bargaining power with third-party payers.
- The suggested educational regimen is worthy of a DPT, and the proposed curriculum includes coursework needed for practice.
- The DPT will help eliminate individuals who are not willing to "go the extra mile" for the profession.
- The DPT will distinguish PTs from other allied health practitioners such as massage therapists, athletic trainers, and kinesiotherapists.
- The content of the suggested DPT curricula does not meet the rigors of medical or dental programs but rather accepts the less stringent standards of regimens for chiropractic, pharmacy, and podiatry.
- Data-based evidence endorsing the DPT is lacking.

Many of the stumbling blocks in this list will be resolved as physical therapy programs work to raise current curricula to the clinical doctorate level. Budget cuts in higher education, faculty credentials, and small applicant pools are among the issues to be addressed. Another consideration is that many medical and law schools now have classes in which women are the majority. This may prove to be a critical issue for a predominantly female profession such as physical therapy because potential applicants may now weigh more carefully the DPT and MD degrees. Conversely, individuals attracted to other nonmedical clinical doctoral degrees, such as pharmacy or chiropractic, may consider physical therapy at the doctoral level more favorably. One thing is certain: regardless of the degree held, PTs must contend with a broader array of issues than ever before.

Perspective of the Practitioner

A key issue for the profession is the conversion by 2020 of licensed PTs with bachelor's and master's degrees to PTs with DPT degrees. Having all PTs hold the same degree designation will reduce the public confusion that arises when the same professionals hold multiple degrees. As PTs become more homogeneous, they will be more easily identified as the primary providers of care for people with movement dysfunction. The ill feeling that might emerge among professionals regarding the value of an academic degree versus the value of experience can thus be diverted.[1]

Through a consensus process, the APTA has developed outcome competencies, a preferred curriculum guide, and a PT evaluation tool (PTET) to assist academic institutions in developing transitional DPT (t-DPT) programs and to aid PTs in preparing their credentials to apply for these programs. The outcome competencies reflect the changes in expectations for entry-level PTs over the past 5 to 10 years. These transitional programs are voluntary and not under the accreditation auspices of the Commission on Accreditation of Physical Therapy Education (CAPTE), as are all other PT and PTA educational programs, and the PTET is not required by all t-DPT programs for admission. These early developmental stages can lead to wide variation in programs, and institutional and regional accreditation committees in higher education must monitor and control quality.[4]

PTs must determine both the cost and the benefit of the t-DPT in their professional development and ability to compete for physical therapy positions. Some considerations include the following:

- PTs nearing retirement are likely to be less interested in the t-DPT degree than more recent graduates of master's degree entry-level programs.
- The degree awarded in t-DPT programs is still an entry-level "equivalency" degree. PTs who already have an entry-level degree may question the value of obtaining another degree to do what they are already licensed to do.
- Many PTs have engaged in professional development over the years, which they may consider at least as valuable as the professional development potential of a t-DPT program.
- Not all entry-level programs award the DPT, and enrollment numbers have decreased in all programs[5]; therefore, the ratio of PTs with bachelor's degrees to those with master's or doctoral degrees is not changing very rapidly. Many programs have only recently made the transition to the master's degree level.
- Employers may be more inclined to favor experience and interpersonal relationship skills over academic credentials, particularly if the degree is perceived as self-serving for the profession or a factor in inflating salaries for PTs.
- Some employers may seek PTs with DPT degrees for marketing purposes, although physicians in some systems may oppose the day-to-day use of the title "Doctor" by nonphysicians.
- The degree the PT holds may not make a difference to patients, who are referred without much choice in which PT treats them.
- The effect of the DPT degree on the referral relationship with physicians, which remains critical to physical therapy practice, is not yet clear.
- The effect, if any, of a t-DPT degree on the long-term career goals of PTs who seek academic careers has not been determined.

The t-DPT is the key to fulfilling the vision of having all PTs hold clinical doctoral degrees. However, without external motivators, such as requiring the DPT for license renewal or basing salary on educational degree, PTs who are already employed and providing quality services may not be convinced the degree is needed.

BOARD CERTIFICATION OF SPECIALISTS

The APTA House of Delegates approved the concept of specialization in PT practice in 1976, and the requirements for certification in advanced clinical competence were approved in 1978. Appointment of the first nine-member American Board of Physical Therapy Specialties (ABPTS) followed shortly thereafter, and subsequently the first specialty council in cardiopulmonary physical therapy was established, which developed criteria and a qualifying examination for this specialty. Over the years, specialty councils have been created for clinical electrophysiology, geriatrics, neurology, orthopedics, pediatrics, and sports physical therapy. The responsibilities of the ABPTS and of each of the specialty councils are listed in Box 3-1.[6]

Perspective of the Profession

The decision to develop a board of specialization for PTs was based on the need to formally recognize PTs with advanced clinical knowledge, experience, and skills in a specialty area of practice so that they could be identified by consumers and the health care community. Specialization is believed to promote (1) the highest possible level of care for individuals seeking physical therapy services in a specialty area and (2) the development of the science and art underlying the specialty.

The specialization program for PTs follows the pattern established for physicians and raises some of the same questions:

- Most physicians seek board certification as specialists; will a similar trend develop for PTs?
- What are the implications if those who choose to specialize come to outnumber those who do not?
- Will PTs identify more with their specialization group than with the general profession?
- Will specialization generate competing professional organizations of PTs as the number certified in each specialty grows (Table 3-1)?

Box **3-1**   Responsibilities of the American Board of Physical Therapy Specialties (ABPTS) and the Specialty Councils

ABPTS

- Develops, implements, and revises policies and procedures related to specialist certification and recertification processes
- Develops the minimum requirements for certification and recertification to be used across all specialty areas and approves the specialty-specific requirements developed by the specialty councils
- Approves and recommends the formation of proposed specialty areas to the APTA House of Delegates and creates those approved
- Oversees the activities of the specialty councils and approves the certification and recertification of qualified specialist candidates

Specialty Council

- Delineates the advanced knowledge, skills, and abilities for their specialty areas and produce the Description of Advanced Clinical Practice/Description of Specialty Practice document
- Determines the academic and clinical requirements for initial certification and recertification
- Screen applicants for eligibility to sit for examinations
- Develops assessment tools (including the certification examination) for initial certification and recertification, in cooperation with the ABPTS testing agency and ABPTS-approved consultants

Table 3-1 | Distribution of Certified Clinical Specialists in Physical Therapy (2003)

Specialty Area	Number of Certified Specialists
Cardiopulmonology	94
Clinical electrophysiology	103
Geriatrics	570
Neurology	374
Orthopedics	2563
Pediatrics	566
Sports	416
Total	4686*

*This number represents about 8% of the more than 60,000 members of the American Physical Therapy Association.

- What impact will increased specialization have on health care costs and quality of care?
- Given the ever-expanding knowledge base, can PTs continue to be generalists?
- Can specialization thrive under managed care, with its emphasis on efficiency?
- Does an alternative mechanism for advancement exist for PTs who are not interested in the administrative career path?

Perspective of the Practitioner

For clinicians, specialization is the process by which they build on their broad base of professional education and practice to develop a greater depth of knowledge and skills related to a particular area of practice. The following eligibility requirements for sitting for the examination to become certified as a PT specialist in any category were modified in 1999[7]:

- Current licensure to practice physical therapy in the United States, District of Columbia, Puerto Rico, or Virgin Islands
- A minimum of 2000 hours of clinical practice in the specialty area, 25% of which must have been within the past 3 years
- Fulfillment of specific requirements unique to each specialty

Board certification is a voluntary process that must be initiated by the PT, who needs to consider several issues when deciding whether to seek this credential. For example, the certification credential is nonrestrictive; it does not prevent others who are not certified from practicing in the area of specialization, and it does not prevent the certified PT from practicing in other areas.[8]

Another consideration is that the certification process is time-consuming and expensive. The specialist is certified for 10 years and then must be recertified to maintain the credential[8]; maintaining board certification, therefore, is a long-term career decision. Board certification in an APTA specialty must be weighed against specialty certifications available through other organizations in disciplines that complement a PT's professional credentials, such as manual therapy, diabetes education, proprioceptive neuromuscular facilitation, lymphedema management, and hand therapy.

According to a survey of certified specialists conducted by the APTA, board certification affects PTs' professional and personal lives.[6] The specialists reported spending more time than nonspecialists in research, teaching, consultation, scholarly productivity, and professional activities. About 40% to 50% said that the certification credential brought them more opportunities for consulting positions, invited presentations, and new jobs, as well as increased professional responsibility. A much higher percentage (about 70%) reported that certification enhanced their prestige and positively affected patient care. More than 80% of certified specialists reported greater personal rewards, including increased self-confidence, a sense of personal achievement, and a more interesting and fulfilling career.[6]

The ABPTS surveyed more than 700 employers of board-certified PTs.[9] Although the responses differed according to the setting, the results generally suggested that both clinical and academic employers believe that having certified specialists on staff is valuable in terms of marketing. About half of the employers paid some of the costs associated with specialization. However, fewer than 50% said that they raised salaries, changed job titles, or increased the authority and responsibility of staff members who became certified specialists, or that they gave hiring preference to board-certified specialists. No more than 50% of the employers agreed that differences could be seen between clinical specialists and nonspecialists in terms of clinical outcomes, ability to manage more complex patient conditions, efficiency, the number of patients referred directly to a particular PT, management positions held, and involvement in roles other than patient care.[9]

These surveys suggest that the personal satisfaction and professional fulfillment derived from achieving board certification are more important to PTs than are external motivators such as a salary increase. Regarding the impact on the quality and outcome of direct patient care, opinion seems to be evenly split between those who believe certification has such an effect and those who do not. This is not surprising, given the complexity of variables other than the PT's credentials that affect patient outcomes.

DIRECT ACCESS ISSUE

Perspective of the Profession

As stated by the APTA, "Direct access is the ability of a physical therapist to provide evaluation and treatment to patients without the need for a physician referral."[10] The public is best served when access is unrestricted.[11] The primary rationale for this position is that direct access eliminates the burden of unnecessary visits to physicians to obtain physical therapy services, which can result in delays and denial of services provided by PTs. The delays in care result in increased costs, decreased functional outcomes, and patient frustration. PTs believe that their extensive education and clinical training make them well qualified to practice without referral, at no increased risk to their patients' health, safety, and welfare.[12]

A sampling of laws that affect direct access (Table 3-2) reflects the variations in restrictions and rules found among states' practice acts.[13] These practice acts are typically discussed in terms of those that place no restrictions on physical therapists in the evaluation and/or treatment of patients without a physician's referral and those that do have restrictions. For example, many jurisdictions allow the PT to perform only an evaluation initially; the patient then must be referred to a physician, who must approve the PT's plan of care before it can be implemented. The differences in the practice acts from state to state reflect the compromises PTs have made, primarily in the 1980s, to reach the profession's goal of direct access in all

Table 3-2 | **Legislation Affecting Direct Access to Physical Therapy in Selected States**

State	Law Enacted	Summary of Provisions
Maryland	1979	• License of the physical therapist (PT) may be revoked if physical therapy is practiced in a manner inconsistent with any written or oral order of a physician, dentist, or podiatrist.
South Dakota	1986	• No restrictions
Iowa	1988	• PT evaluation and treatment may be provided with or without a referral from a physician, podiatric physician, dentist, or chiropractor; however, a hospital may require that PT evaluation and treatment provided in the hospital be performed only after prior review and authorization by a member of the hospital's medical staff.
		• PTs are prohibited from practicing operative surgery and osteopathic or chiropractic manipulation; also, they may not administer or prescribe drugs or medicines.
New Mexico	1989	• PTs shall not accept a patient for treatment without an existing medical diagnosis for the specific medical or physical problem; this diagnosis must be made by a licensed primary care provider, except for children in special education programs and for acute care within the scope of physical therapy practice.
		• PTs must update the patient's primary health care provider on the physical therapy diagnosis and plan of treatment every 60 days unless otherwise directed by the primary care provider.
Florida	1992	• PT must refer the patient or consult with a health care practitioner if the patient's condition is outside the scope of physical therapy practice.
		• If physical therapy treatment is required for longer than 21 days for a condition not previously assessed by a practitioner of record, the PT must arrange to work with a practitioner of record, who will review and sign the plan.
		• PTs may not implement a plan of treatment for patients in acute care settings, including hospitals, ambulatory surgical centers, and mobile surgical facilities.
Rhode Island	1992	• PTs must disclose to the patient in writing the scope and limitations of the practice of physical therapy and must obtain their consent to treatment in writing.
		• PTs must refer the patient to a doctor of medicine, osteopathy, dentistry, podiatry, or chiropractic within 90 days after treatment begins (unless the treatment has concluded).
		• PTs must have 1 year clinical experience to practice without referral.

jurisdictions. Efforts to achieve the right to direct access continue in states that do not yet have it.

In an effort to explain the differences in practice acts that have emerged from efforts to obtain direct access, Taylor and Domholdt[14] surveyed APTA chapter presidents about the process of modifying physical therapy practice acts and found that patients, state physical therapy associations, home health and extended care facilities, and some insurance companies openly supported direct access to PTs. Groups that expressed opposition included hospital associations, some insurance companies, medical associations, physicians, and chiropractors, as well as physical therapists themselves. In some states, the opposition to direct access included groups who supported it in other states.

Objections to direct access included (1) the belief that education of PTs was not sufficient to allow them to serve as initial contacts for entry into the health care system; (2) the risk that serious medical problems might be missed in systems other than the musculoskeletal system; and (3) the fear that increasing the autonomy of PTs would shift them to private practice and create staffing shortages in hospitals.[14] Despite these objections, Durant, Lord, and Domholdt[15] found that 83% of outpatients in Indiana would seek PTs through direct access if they were allowed to do so.

Domholdt and Durchholz[16] addressed the issue of the impact of direct access in states where it is permitted by conducting a study of PTs in North Carolina, Nevada, and Utah. In these states, 44% of PTs had practiced through direct access. Those who did estimated that about 10.3% of their caseloads was composed of patients seen without a physician's referral; 40% of those patients were referred to physicians.

Reasons PTs gave for not practicing through direct access included prohibitive policies by employers that prevented direct access practice; the requirement by third-party payers of a physician referral for reimbursement of services; and the PT's personal preference to treat by referral only, perhaps because the PT was employed by a physician or feared that physicians would no longer refer.

Domholdt and Durchholz suggested that the results of their study be considered cautiously because the sample of PTs was small. However, they also stated that the reasons for practicing only by referral may reflect "the inertia of therapists used to practicing in a more dependent mode."[16]

The APTA has identified the primary barrier to direct access as the Medicare Part B requirement that beneficiaries get a physician's referral for physical therapy to obtain coverage of these services. The APTA has targeted this rule for elimination, stating its position thus:

> The American Physical Therapy Association (APTA) strongly supports the ability of licensed physical therapists to evaluate, diagnose, and treat beneficiaries requiring outpatient physical therapy services under Part B of the Medicare program, without a physician referral. The physician referral is unnecessary and limits access to timely and medically necessary physical therapists' services.[6]

Whether taking the direct access issue to the federal level will succeed remains to be seen. However, if Part B is successfully revised, private insurers probably will follow Medicare's lead and amend their own regulations.

Perspective of the Practitioner

Although the rationale for direct access is clear from the perspectives of the patient and the profession, the reasons PTs practice with or without referral in their daily work require further exploration. For some PTs, the issue may not be important because they are comfortable with and accustomed to their current referral relationships with physicians; others who practice through referral may not feel that they have faced any professional limitations with the arrangement. In particular, PTs employed by health care systems with institutional regulations covering referral of both inpatients and outpatients may lack a sense of urgency about this issue. Some PTs, especially those in independent practices, may want more opportunity to market and provide their services directly to patients, but they may have no choice but to meet reimbursement criteria for referral in order to be paid.

Another potential obstacle for some PTs is their reluctance to accept total responsibility for systems screening of patients who have not seen a physician. The acquisition and interpretation of laboratory, radiographic, and other imaging tests are beyond the scope of practice of physical therapists. Although PTs currently are responsible for screening all systems as part of the history taking and examination of each patient, thoroughness in this screening in some patients may be challenging without the support of medical diagnostics. With patients who have no access to physicians, such diagnostic testing may be even more important in the screening of systems (other than the neuromusculoskeletal system) that typically are not considered the purview of PTs. Another challenge for the PT may be determining a course of action when the history and examination reveal a need for referral to a physician although the patient does not have a doctor or cannot afford one.

Finally, should the rule on referral from a physician be eliminated, it remains to be seen what Medicare administrative and documentation requirements may result.

PHYSICAL THERAPIST ASSISTANTS

Perspective of the Profession

The definition of physical therapy found in the APTA's *Guide to Physical Therapist Practice* delineates the relationship between the PT and the PTA[17]:

> Physical therapy is defined as the care and service provided by or under the direction and supervision of a physical therapist. Physical therapists are the only professionals who provide physical therapy. Physical therapist assistants—under the direction and supervision of the physical therapist—are the only paraprofessionals who assist in the provision of physical therapy interventions.
>
> APTA therefore recommends that federal and state government agencies and other third-party payers require physical therapy to be provided only by a physical therapist or under the direction and supervision of a physical therapist. Examination, evaluation, diagnosis, and prognosis should be represented and reimbursed as physical therapy only when they are performed by a physical therapist. Intervention should be represented and reimbursed as physical therapy only when performed by a physical therapist or by a physical therapist assistant under the direction and supervision of a physical therapist.

The PTA is a technically educated health care provider who assists the PT in the provision of physical therapy. In the contemporary provision of physical therapy services, the PT is considered the professional practitioner of physical therapy, and the PTA, educated at the technical level, is considered the paraprofessional.[18]

These definitions specify the exclusivity of the term *physical therapy* (often phrased as, "It's only physical therapy if a physical therapist does it") and then extend the term's use to include services provided by PTAs under the direction and supervision of the PT. The exclusivity issue has proved to be an important topic, one related to the *Current Procedural Terminology* (CPT) billing codes used by health care professionals. The problem arises when billing codes commonly used by physical therapists are referred to as "Physical Therapy" although the person providing the care for which a bill is submitted is not a physical therapist.

The definitions also make it clear that services provided by PTAs constitute physical therapy only if performed under the supervision and direction of a PT and that PTAs are the only paraprofessionals who may perform physical therapy services. State statutes that control the direction and supervision of support personnel affect the implementation of the APTA definitions, and rules for reimbursement may vary from insurer to insurer and intermediary to intermediary. Therefore adoption of these definitions by jurisdictions, and particularly by Medicare, is essential to the clarification of the PTA's role.

History

The position of PTA was created by the APTA House of Delegates in 1966, prompted by a need for support personnel in the profession. In 1973 the affiliate membership category was created, allowing PTAs to become members of the APTA and to be represented in the House of Delegates, where each elected PTA had half a vote. In 1998 the affiliate members (PTAs) and the active members (PTs) were divided into separate governing groups. Affiliate members now make up the National Assembly of Physical Therapist Assistants, and PTs comprise the American College of Physical Therapists.[19]

During this time legislation was passed in many jurisdictions to license PTAs, and these efforts continue today. The statutory rules that determine the supervisory relationship of the PT over the PTA vary, perhaps as a result of the staffing needs in each jurisdiction as the laws were developed. For instance, in rural states, which may have a significant shortage of PTs, the rules may allow less restrictive supervision of the PTA in order to meet the need for physical therapy services in sparsely populated areas (see Chapter 10).

Killen[20] saw the initial impetus for the development of the PTA position as a response to the shortage of physical therapy personnel in the 1960s. This shortage was primarily the result of implementation of the Medicare program, which increased the demand for rehabilitation services for the elderly and others with chronic conditions. The author suggested that because PTs had been rejecting the professional responsibilities of supervision, administration, education, and research, they were reluctant to give up many duties that support personnel could perform. In other words, PTs did not want to give up or share direct patient care responsibilities because they thought the result would be desk work that separated them from the hands-on care that was the heart of their profession.

A 1971 study by Watts[21] reflected the professional mood of the times regarding the PTA. As yet, little consensus had been reached, and a great deal of uneasiness about relinquishing tasks to PTAs persisted, although physical therapists were facing the challenge of maintaining quality of care while keeping the cost of services as low as possible.

Watts suggested that PTs ask themselves three questions when considering the use of support personnel[21]:
1. Does the PT perform some tasks that could be done as well or better by others?
2. Does the PT perform some tasks that could be done as well by others most of the time but might result on relatively rare (and perhaps unpredictable) occasions in complications that a less well-trained individual could not handle?

3. Does the PT perform some tasks that others would perform less well but, as a result of the increase in staffing, more often, in the best interest of society?

Watts cautioned that the answers to these questions should not lead to the potentially dangerous practice of classifying tasks as routinely belonging to support personnel. The procedures PTs perform may be simple or complex, depending on the circumstances. Therefore, an intentional overlap of competence, with some flexibility, must exist between PTs and PTAs because of the individual abilities of each, and some specialization is required at both levels. In other words, a PT is not a super-PTA, and a PTA is not a partly trained PT. Watts predicted that direct patient care would always be a substantial part of the work of PTs, but that they would work with larger numbers of patients for less time. As a result, the PTA would have to be the eyes, ears, and fingertips of the PT in a shared responsibility for patient care that demands a high degree of interdependence.[22] More than 30 years later, PTs still might ask themselves Watts's three questions about the use of support personnel.

Recent Studies

Although the use of PTAs and other support personnel has become more common-place, controversy persists. In 1999 Figueroa-Soto et al.[22] published a study of PTs in Pennsylvania in which subjects were asked to identify the unique contributions of physical therapy to patient care and to report which of these duties were delegated. Twenty-six tasks were identified as contributions unique to physical therapy. A task that was delegated by 30% or more of the subjects was designated "most delegated." Twenty-three of the tasks fell into this category. The top 11 ranked tasks were considered the contributions most identifiably unique to physical therapy. The percentage of PTs who delegated these tasks to PTAs ranged from 21% to 58%, and 37% to 88% of the study participants indicated that they supervised those delegated tasks by observing or assisting. Figueroa-Soto et al. concluded that the tasks named in the study were unique to the profession of physical therapy but not to PTs, because PTAs are such an integral part of the delivery of patient care and many tasks are delegated to them. They also found that the role of the PTA appeared to be expanding.[22]

About the same time, Robinson and colleagues conducted two studies, one involving PTs and the other PTAs, to determine the two groups' perceptions of the documented roles of the PTA.[23,24] Professional documents, such as the CAPTE criteria for PTA programs and the policies of the APTA House of Delegates, as well as other research studies, were used to develop the survey items. For analysis purposes, the roles of the PTA were categorized as evaluation activities, treatment planning, treatment implementation, and administrative roles. Although the survey used the term "evaluation," the questions actually addressed patient examination items, such as "perform joint range of motion [ROM] tests" and "assess muscle tone," which are appropriate PTA tasks. At the conclusion of the two studies, the results were compared.

The perceptions of the PTs and the PTAs differed on 9 of the 24 items in the "evaluation" category; on four of the 14 items in the treatment planning category; on 2 of the 25 items in the treatment implementation category; and on 5 of the 15 items in the administrative roles category. Some of the differences within each group and between the two groups regarding evaluation were thought to be related to a revision of the CAPTE criteria, occurring shortly after the studies. These new criteria significantly expanded the list of assessments in which PTAs were to become competent and may have had some influence on the thinking of the respondents. In treatment planning, the studies' results indicated that PTAs prefer to work under plans of care that leave some decision making in their hands, whereas PTs prefer to design a more prescriptive plans of care for PTAs to implement. The responses to the administrative roles of the PTA in treatment implementation suggested that both PTs and PTAs thought more roles were documented than actually was the case. Finally, the lack of consensus on these roles implied that more study was required on the issue of tasks that involve developing policies and procedures, selecting capital equipment, planning staff development, and developing quality assurance and space management programs.

These studies show that consensus has not yet been reached on who does what in physical therapy, and the issue may continue to be in flux because of the complicated environments in which PTs and PTAs work. These individual but overlapping environments pose different challenges to the delicate balance between staffing levels that allow quality service and the need to hold down costs—the twin controlling factors in contemporary health care.

Other Issues

As the physical therapy profession continues to evolve, so will the role of the PTA. Among the issues that must be resolved are the following:

- Should the educational level of the PTA be raised,[25] and will the responsibilities of the PTA change as the DPT becomes the norm (Box 3-2)?
- Changes in the demand for PTAs are closely connected to staffing needs, which are secondarily connected to reimbursement policies. (For example, in an employment survey conducted by the APTA in the fall of 2001, the percentage of PTAs who were not working but wanted to had dropped to 3.9% from 6.5% the year before. Of those who were not employed, 15.2% said it was at least partly because of salary reductions or because the number of hours worked was so high, they terminated their positions. These employment trends are linked to policies resulting from the Balanced Budget Act of 1997, which led some employers to alter staffing patterns in their efforts to reduce costs related to changes in Medicare that were part of this act.[26])
- Will direct access to physical therapy result in greater delegation of routine tasks as PTs take on greater responsibility for patients without physician referral?

Perspective of the Practitioner

Watts's warning about the "dangerous practice of classifying tasks as routinely belonging to supportive personnel"[21] remains potent today. In the complex, interdependent relationship between PTs and PTAs, nothing can replace the independent judgment of PTs in delegating responsibility. Watts's[21] list of five points to consider before deciding to delegate care remains helpful:

1. *Predictability of consequences:* How uncertain is the situation? How confident can the decision maker be in predicting the consequences of action?
2. *Stability of the situation:* How much and how quickly is change likely to occur in the factors on which decisions are based?
3. *Observability of basic indicators:* How difficult is it to elicit the phenomena on which decisions are based? How easy are these phenomena to perceive?
4. *Ambiguity of basic indicators:* How difficult are the key phenomena to interpret? How easily might they be confused with other phenomena?
5. *Criticality of results:* How serious are the consequences of a poor choice of goals or method?

Box 3-2   Evaluative Criteria for Physical Therapist Assistant Programs

Communication

3.3.2.1. Communicates verbally and nonverbally with the patient, the physical therapist, health care delivery personnel, and others in an effective, appropriate, and capable manner

Individual and Cultural Differences

3.3.2.2. Recognizes individual and cultural differences and responds appropriately in all aspects of physical therapy services

Behavior and Conduct

3.3.2.3. Exhibits conduct that reflects a commitment to meeting the expectations of members of society receiving health care services

3.3.2.4. Exhibits conduct that reflects a commitment to meeting the expectations of members of the profession of physical therapy

3.3.2.5. Exhibits conduct that reflects practice standards that are legal, ethical, and safe

Plan of Care

3.3.2.6. Communicates an understanding of the plan of care developed by the physical therapist to achieve short- and long-term goals and intended outcomes

3.3.2.7. Demonstrates competence in the implementation of selected components of interventions identified in the plan of care established by the physical therapist

3.3.2.8. Demonstrates competency in the performance of components of data collection skills essential for carrying out the plan of care

3.3.2.9. Adjusts interventions within the plan of care established by the physical therapist in response to the patient's clinical indications and reports such adjustments to the supervising physical therapist

3.3.2.10. Recognizes when intervention should not be provided because of changes in the patient's status and reports this to the supervising physical therapist

3.3.2.11. Reports any changes in the patient's status to the supervising physical therapist

3.3.2.12. Recognizes when performance of an intervention is beyond the skill level appropriate for a physical therapist assistant and initiates clarification with the physical therapist

3.3.2.13. Participates in the education of patients and caregivers as directed by the supervising physical therapist

3.3.2.14. Provides patient-related instruction to patients, family members, and caregivers to achieve patient outcomes based on the plan of care established by the physical therapist

3.3.2.15. Takes appropriate action in an emergency

3.3.2.16. Completes thorough, accurate, logical, concise, timely, and legible documentation that follows guidelines and specific documentation formats required by state practice acts, regulatory agencies, and the practice setting

3.3.2.17. Participates in discharge planning and follow-up as directed by the supervising physical therapist

3.3.2.18. Reads and understands the health care literature

Education

3.3.2.19. Under the direction and supervision of the physical therapist, instructs other members of the health care team using established techniques, programs, and instructional materials commensurate with the learning characteristics of the audience

3.3.2.20. Educates others about the role of the physical therapist assistant

Administration

3.3.2.21. Interacts with other members of the health care team in patient care and nonpatient care activities

Box 3-2   Evaluative Criteria for Physical Therapist Assistant Programs—cont'd

Administration (cont'd)

3.3.2.22. Provides accurate and timely information for billing and reimbursement purposes

3.3.2.23. Can describe aspects of the organizational planning and operation of the physical therapy service

3.3.2.24. Participates in performance improvement activities (quality assurance)

Social Responsibility

3.3.2.25. Demonstrates a commitment to meeting the needs of patients and consumers

3.3.2.26. Demonstrates an awareness of social responsibility, citizenship, and advocacy, including participation in community and service organizations and activities

Career Development

3.3.2.27 Identifies career development and lifelong learning opportunities

3.3.2.28 Recognizes the role of the physical therapist assistant in the clinical education of physical therapist assistant students

From the Commission on Accreditation of Physical Therapy Education. *Evaluative criteria for accreditation of education programs for the preparation of physical therapist assistants.* Retrieved November 11, 2003, at http://www.apta.org/AM/Template/cfm?Section=Program_Info&TEMPLATE=/CM/ContentDisplay.cfm&CONTENTID=22223

PTs may not always have a choice about the ratio of PTs to PTAs in their work setting, or their choices may result in less than satisfactory relationships in terms of interdependency. The following are some examples of staffing patterns:

- A PT is partnered with one PTA, and the two share responsibility for an assigned patient load.
- PTAs significantly outnumber PTs; the PT therefore delegates care to more than one PTA.
- PTs significantly outnumber PTAs. The PTAs, therefore, function in one of two ways: (1) each PTA has an independent personal caseload, made up of patients who were evaluated by one or more PTs and then transferred to the PTA for implementation of patient care; or (2) the PTA works with several PTs, implementing the plans of care with the PTs.
- The staff includes no PTAs; PTs provide all direct patient care.

Except in the partnership model, the strong interdependence between the PT and the PTA may be compromised; alternatively, the norm may be that specific tasks are always assigned to the PTA. PTs may need to address these staffing patterns in terms of quality of care and the reduction of risks to patients receiving physical therapy. At the same time, if external influences are discouraging the use of support personnel, PTs may be unable to assume their responsibilities in roles other than direct patient care and unable to focus on the unique patient skills that cannot be delegated because they are performing *all* patient care tasks.

THE GUIDE—AN EXTRAORDINARY ACHIEVEMENT

In the 1990s the Florida Physical Therapy Association was asked by the state's agency for health care administration to help develop practice parameters for individuals with low back pain. Recognizing that these parameters needed to be based on national rather than statewide collaboration, the Florida Physical Therapy Association asked the APTA to join the project, which was expanded to include other areas. Contributions from more than 600 experts in various fields were fine-tuned and integrated, and in 1997 the *Guide to Physical Therapist Practice* was published.[27] (Its current title is the *Interactive Guide to Physical Therapist Practice with Catalog of Tests and Measures*.[17]) This publication has come to be known simply as "the *Guide*."

Those in the profession recognized that before they could envision where the practice of physical therapy is headed, they had to know where it currently stands. The *Guide* has helped ground the profession in a central document that serves as the starting point for the APTA research agenda and the policies that steer the profession in meeting its vision (see A Vision for the Future, page 45).

Perspective of the Profession

The *Guide* remains a resource for health care policy makers. It also serves as a major resource for PTs in a variety of roles, including students. PTs in clinical practice may use the *Guide* for individual decision making, continuous quality-improvement programs, and outcome studies. Health care administrators, managed-care providers, and third-party payers may refer to the *Guide* in deciding on the provision and payment of physical therapy services. Accreditation criteria and the APTA research agenda have been modified to make them consistent with the terminology and purpose of the *Guide*.

The *Guide* serves the following purposes in the profession[2]:
- Describes PT practice in general
- Describes the roles of PTs in primary, secondary, and tertiary care; prevention; and promotion of health, wellness, and fitness
- Describes the settings in which PTs practice
- Standardizes the terminology used in and related to PT practice
- Establishes the tests and measures, as well as interventions, used in PT practice
- Delineates preferred-practice patterns to help PTs accomplish the following[17]:
  - Improve the quality of care
  - Enhance the positive outcomes of physical therapy services
  - Enhance patient satisfaction
  - Promote appropriate use of health care services
  - Increase efficiency and reduce unwarranted variation in the provision of services
  - Diminish the economic burden of disablement through prevention of poor health practices and promotion of health, wellness, and fitness initiatives

Because the *Guide* is the result of a consensus process, it does not include specific recommended plans of care, protocols, or clinical guidelines, which traditionally are based on a comprehensive search and systematic evaluation of peer-reviewed literature. Rather, the *Guide* encompasses the breadth of practice through practice patterns that include options for care rather than standards of care. Two primary purposes of the *Guide* are to delineate the practice patterns and to define the role of the PT in the prevention of illness and the promotion of health, wellness, and fitness.

Practice Patterns

The practice patterns are presented in Box 3-3[17]; each pattern includes the components listed in Table 3-3.[17]

Box **3-3**   Physical Therapy Practice Patterns

Musculoskeletal	Neuromuscular	Cardiovascular Pulmonary	Integumentary
4A: Primary Prevention/Risk Reduction for Skeletal Demineralization	5A: Primary Prevention/Risk Reduction for Loss of Balance and Falling	6A: Primary Prevention/Risk Reduction for Cardiovascular/ Pulmonary Disorders	7A: Primary Prevention/Risk Reduction for Integumentary Disorders
4B: Impaired Posture	5B: Impaired Neuromotor Development	6B: Impaired Aerobic Capacity/ Endurance Associated With Deconditioning	7B: Impaired Integumentary Integrity Associated With Superficial Skin Involvement
4C: Impaired Muscle Performance	5C: Impaired Motor Function and Sensory Integrity Associated With Nonprogressive Disorders of the Central Nervous System— Congenital Origin or Acquired in Infancy or Childhood	6C: Impaired Ventilation, Respiration/Gas Exchange, and Aerobic Capacity/ Endurance Associated With Airway Clearance Dysfunction	7C: Impaired Integumentary Integrity Associated With Partial-Thickness Skin Involvement and Scar Formation
4D: Impaired Joint Mobility, Motor Function, Muscle Performance, and Range of Motion Associated With Connective Tissue Dysfunction			7D: Impaired Integumentary Integrity Associated With Full-Thickness Skin Involvement and Scar Formation
4E: Impaired Joint Mobility, Motor Function, Muscle Performance, and Range of Motion Associated With Localized Inflammation	5D: Impaired Motor Function and Sensory Integrity Associated With Nonprogressive Disorders of the Central Nervous System— Acquired in Adolescence or Adulthood	6D: Impaired Aerobic Capacity/ Endurance Associated With Cardiovascular Pump Dysfunction or Failure	7E: Impaired Integumentary Integrity Associated With Skin Involvement Extending Into Fascia, Muscle, or Bone and Scar Formation
4F: Impaired Joint Mobility, Motor Function, Muscle Performance, Range of Motion, and Reflex Integrity Associated With Spinal Disorders	5E: Impaired Motor Function and Sensory Integrity Associated With Progressive Disorders of the Central Nervous System	6E: Impaired Ventilation and Respiration/Gas Exchange Associated With Ventilatory Pump Dysfunction or Failure	
4G: Impaired Joint Mobility, Muscle Performance, and Range of Motion Associated With Fracture	5F: Impaired Peripheral Nerve Integrity and	6F: Impaired Ventilation and Respiration/Gas Exchange Associated With	
4H: Impaired Joint Mobility, Motor Function, Muscle Performance, and Range of Motion			

Box **3-3**   **PHYSICAL THERAPY PRACTICE PATTERNS—CONT'D**

Musculoskeletal	Neuromuscular	Cardiovascular Pulmonary	Integumentary
Associated With Joint Arthroplasty	Muscle Performance Associated With Peripheral Nerve Injury	Respiratory Failure	
4I: Impaired Joint Mobility, Motor Function, Muscle Performance, and Range of Motion Associated With Bony or Soft Tissue Surgery	5G: Impaired Motor Function and Sensory Integrity Associated With Acute or Chronic Polyneuropathies	6G: Impaired Ventilation, Respiration/Gas Exchange, and Aerobic Capacity/ Endurance Associated With Respiratory Failure in the Neonate	
4J: Impaired Motor Function, Muscle Performance, Range of Motion, Gait, Locomotion, and Balance Associated With Amputation	5H: Impaired Motor Function, Peripheral Nerve Integrity, and Sensory Integrity Associated With Nonprogressive Disorders of the Spinal Cord	6H: Impaired Circulation and Anthropometric Dimensions Associated With Lymphatic System Disorders	
	5I: Impaired Arousal, Range of Motion, and Motor Control Associated With Coma, Near Coma, or Vegetative State		

From American Physical Therapy Association. *Interactive guide to physical therapist practice with catalog of tests and measures* (version 1.0). Alexandria, Va: The Association. This material is copyrighted, and any further reproduction or distribution is prohibited.

The labels of the practice patterns serve as PT diagnoses, because they identify the impact of a condition on function at the level of the system (especially the movement system) and at the level of the whole person, which is where the PT's responsibility lies—to restore function in a disablement model. However, because PTs work in the medical model, it is important to identify the links between the disablement model and the medical model and between medical and physical therapy diagnoses (Figure 3-1).[17]

The dotted box in Figure 3-1 shows the scope of physical therapy practice, which extends into the medical model at one end. This extension demands that PTs relate to physicians at the level of disease or injury, where physicians' expertise lies. The medical diagnosis addresses the cause of the patient's pathologic condition, and the medical interventions (primarily medications and surgical procedures) that address those causes. At the opposite end of the box, the scope of physical therapy practice extends into the realm of disability; this demands that PTs consider the broader social contexts of patients with disabilities. Responsibility for aiding

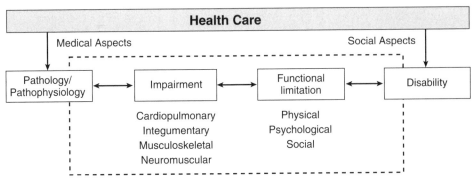

Figure 3-1. Physical therapy scope of practice in the continuum of health care services and the context of the disablement model. *(Modified from Guccione AA. Physical therapy diagnosis and the relationship between impairments and function. Phys Ther 1991;71:499-504.)*

Table 3-3 | **Components of a Practice Pattern**

Component	*Description*
Diagnostic classification	Criteria used to determine whether a patient will be included in or excluded from a pattern based on examination findings of impairments, functional limitations, or disabilities
ICD-9-CM codes	The International Classification of Diseases codes that may relate to the practice pattern; they are intended for information only and are not used for billing or record keeping purposes
Examination	Description of the history, systems review, and tests and measures that generate data used by the physical therapist to help confirm classification of the patient/client in the practice pattern
Evaluation, diagnosis, and prognosis	Processes that provide information on the potential number of visits and on factors that may require a new episode of care or may modify the frequency of visits or the duration of episodes
Intervention	List of treatments that may be used for patients/clients classified into the practice pattern
Reexamination, outcomes, and termination	Processes that determine when reexamination is indicated; measure global outcomes of physical therapy services in eight domains*; and establish criteria for termination of physical therapy services

*The eight outcome domains are pathology/pathophysiology, impairments, functional limitations, disabilities, risk reduction/prevention, health, wellness, and fitness, societal resources, and patient/client satisfaction.

disabled people is part of the role of social workers and case managers at the individual level and policy makers at the broader societal level. PTs may extend their practice into this end of the disablement model by serving as advocates for people with disabilities, particularly in the development of public policy related to the rights of people with disabilities and their participation in society.

Consistent with this scope of practice, the practice patterns are organized into categories (diagnoses); these focus on impairments associated with broad categories of disease and injury in the major body systems that most demand the attention of PTs.

Conditions across the life span are included in each pattern. With the intent of being as inclusive as possible, the practice patterns provide a great deal of information related to all tests, measures, anticipated goals, and interventions that may be appropriate for people with the conditions described in each pattern. Although the patterns classify physical therapy diagnoses into separate groups, considerable repetition may be seen in each pattern; this is to be expected, because PTs use the same patient/client management process regardless of the diagnosis.

This consistency of expectations in the practice patterns and the classifications may be valuable as PTs work with third-party payers to obtain reimbursement approval for plans of care. The APTA has distributed the *Guide* to all its members and to many third-party payers. Efforts to encourage incorporation of the *Guide*, particularly the terminology, into physical therapy practice and to promote its use by third-party payers in their decision making continue, even as the document itself evolves.

The *Guide* has been a major step in identifying the common approach to patient/client management in physical therapy, but at this stage it is about preferences and delineations. A great deal of work needs to be done. For instance, the current edition of the *Guide* presents studies on the validity and reliability of some of the tests and measures, but it does not provide any agreed-upon recommendations regarding which of these may be most valuable. The efficacy of the physical therapy interventions is not addressed at all in the latest edition of the *Guide*. However, to fill this gap the APTA has undertaken a grass-roots initiative, Hooked on Evidence, a Web-based tool to access evidenced-based reviews of physical therapy studies.

Broadening the Practice Context

In addition to establishing the disablement model as the guiding principle in the practice patterns, the *Guide* places the scope of PT practice in the broader environmental context, which includes other factors that influence impairments and functional limitations, such as biological and demographic characteristics, comorbidities, and psychological attributes (Figure 3-2).[17] PTs' scope of practice is affected by medical practice and, perhaps more important, by the prevention of illness and the promotion of health and wellness.

There are three types of prevention[17]:

- *Primary prevention* is the prevention of disease in a susceptible or potentially susceptible population through specific measures, such as general health promotion efforts (e.g., vaccination of health care workers for hepatitis B).
- *Secondary prevention* involves efforts to shorten the duration of illness, ameliorate the severity of disease, and reduce sequelae through early diagnosis and prompt intervention (e.g., the use of mammograms and other screening techniques for early detection of cancer).
- *Tertiary prevention* is characterized by efforts to reduce the degree of disability and to promote rehabilitation and restoration of function in patients with chronic and irreversible diseases. In the diagnostic process, the PT identifies risk factors for disability that may exist independently of the disease or injury (e.g., interdisciplinary rehabilitation for individuals with traumatic head injury).

PTs are most commonly involved, and their roles are most straightforward, in tertiary and secondary prevention. PTs intervene to increase the functional activity of individuals with reversible postsurgical or acute injuries (secondary prevention) and participate in traditional rehabilitation (tertiary prevention).

The role of PTs in primary prevention is less evident, but PTs have a definite place in patient/client management of people beyond the traditional model, as is reflected

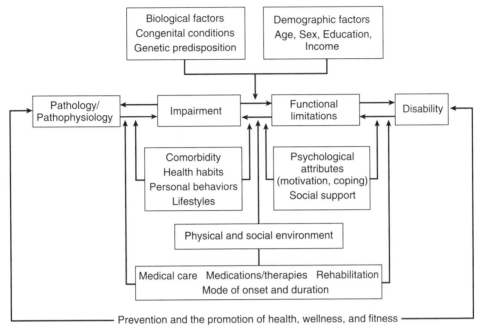

Figure 3-2. Expanded scope of practice of the physical therapist. *(Modified from Guccione AA. Arthritis and the process of disablement. Phys Ther 1994;74:410.)*

in the expanded model of disablement (see Figure 3-2). As defined by the *Guide,*[17] the broadened scope of physical therapy practice includes addressing risk (identifying risk factors and behaviors that may impede optimal functioning) and providing the following services to prevent illness and to promote health, wellness, and fitness:

- Prevention services that forestall functional decline and the need for more intense care
- Timely and appropriate screening, examination, evaluation, diagnosis, prognosis, and intervention to reduce or eliminate the need for costlier forms of care and possibly to shorten or even eliminate institutional stays
- Promotion of health, wellness, and fitness initiatives, including education and services that prompt the public to engage in healthy behaviors

The *Guide* defines an *episode* of physical therapy prevention as a series of occasional clinical, educational, and administrative services related to the prevention of illness; the promotion of health, wellness, and fitness; and the preservation of optimal function. No defined number or range of visits is given for this type of care. However, as a vital part of the practice of physical therapy, such episodes may include three primary programs[17]: (1) prevention services; (2) programs that promote health, wellness, and fitness; and (3) programs for maintenance of function.

Although many PTs may participate in such formalized programs, particularly for groups of patients in the maintenance of function, they less commonly engage in such programs for the general public. One reason may be that this kind of work constitutes a lucrative business for licensed and unlicensed providers outside the health care setting. For example, personal trainers, athletic trainers, and exercise physiologists may be employed by gyms and training centers to provide fitness programs. In the health care system, nurses or public health professionals typically assume primary responsibility for health and wellness programs, particularly those with a strong educational focus. It appears appropriate that PTs include these responsibilities among their roles, but where and how PTs fit into the health/wellness/fitness industry remains to be determined, although these expanded roles appear repeatedly in the *Guide*.

These roles also appear in the *Guide* in the risk reduction/prevention and health/wellness/fitness domains (as well as elsewhere), because physical therapy services affect the outcomes of these interventions.[17]

Perspective of the Practitioner

The risk reduction/prevention role of the PT in patient/client management seems less formalized than other professional responsibilities. Many PTs may not commonly include information on behaviors that are health risks as part of the history and systems screening. For instance, measuring blood pressure in all patients to identify or monitor hypertension or discussing the risks of smoking with patients who smoke or asking a female patient when she last had a Papanicolaou (PAP) smear may not be routine procedures during the history taking and examination.

Particularly as direct access for patients advances, PTs may want to reconsider their responsibilities for risk identification and counseling in the absence of physicians. However, PTs even now have a responsibility to explore health risks that may not appear to have a direct relationship to physical therapy. PTs spend lots of time with patients on an extended basis, which gives them more opportunity than many other health professionals to address health risk behaviors. If every PT prevented just one major illness or injury a month by addressing these health risks in each patient, the impact on mortality rates in the United States might be impressive (Box 3-4).

THE APTA AND POLITICAL ACTION

Perspective of the Profession

To transform its vision into reality, the APTA, like any professional group, must participate in the political process. The organization engages in two activities: political action committees (PACs) and lobbying.

Political Action Committees

PACs are organized to raise and spend money to elect or defeat political candidates. PACs have existed since 1944, when the Congress of Industrial Organizations (CIO) formed the first one to raise money for the reelection of President Franklin D. Roosevelt.[28] Since 1975 PACs have had to register with and have been monitored by the Federal Election Commission (FEC), which regulates federal elections and discloses campaign finance information. The FEC enforces the provisions of related laws, such as limits and prohibitions on contributions, and oversees public funding of presidential elections.[29] For example, a PAC's money must come from voluntary contributions from individuals or from members of an organization; it may not be taken from the general funds of an organization because these are legally considered separate funds. PACs also are limited in the amount of money they can contribute. Currently they may contribute up to $5,000 to a political candidate per election, or $15,000 to any national party committee, or $5,000 to another PAC.[29]

Box 3-4   **HEALTH RISK DISCUSSION POINTS FOR CLIENT EDUCATION**

Important Factors that Affect Health*

Physical activity
Overweight and obesity
Tobacco use
Substance abuse
Responsible sexual behavior
Mental health
Injury and violence
Environmental quality
Immunization
Access to health care

Ten Leading Causes of Death in the United States (2002)†

Heart disease
Cancer
Stroke
Chronic lower respiratory disease
Accidents
Diabetes
Pneumonia/influenza
Alzheimer's disease
Nephritis, nephrotic syndrome, nephrosis
Septicemia

---

*From Healthy People 2010. *Leading health indicators.* Retrieved November 11, 2003, at
http://www.healthypeople.gov/LHI/
†From Centers for Disease Control and Prevention. *Fastats.* Retrieved November 11, 2003, at
http://www.cdc.gov/nchs/fastats/lcod.htm

The Physical Therapy Political Action Committee (PT-PAC) states that its purpose is to "ensure that physical therapy maintains a forceful voice in the halls of Congress."[30] It promotes the profession of physical therapy by supporting members of Congress who are friends of the physical therapy profession."[30] In the 1997-1998 election cycle, PT-PAC raised more than $800,000 through contributions and other fund-raising activities. Fifty-two percent of the money went to Republicans, and the rest was distributed to Democrats campaigning for election.[31]

Members of PT-PAC are appointed by the APTA Board of Directors. Their tasks, as presented on their Web page, are "to raise funds to contribute to campaigns of candidates for national and state office, with attention to PTs as candidates for public office, and to encourage and facilitate APTA member participation in the political process."[32]

Lobbying

Lobbyists are employed by an organization to represent the group to elected legislators. Lobbyists represent the organization's interests and advance its legislative agenda. The vision of the APTA depends on the efforts of lobbyists at the federal and state levels, particularly as they work with grassroots member networks to achieve the legislative goals established by the organization.

For example, in a state in which PTs want to revise the physical therapy practice act, a lobbyist may be responsible for identifying members of the legislature who would sponsor the bills necessary to change the statutes. All members of the state's APTA chapter might then be called upon as constituents to contact their state representatives and senators to ask for their support of these bills. These efforts are an important responsibility, one that includes educating legislators about the profession and its importance in promoting the health of the citizens they represent.

Perspective of the Practitioner

Whether to support PT-PAC or any other PAC is an important decision for PTs. Without the additional financial support of PTs, the influence of the APTA on legislative decisions would be nonexistent. Supporting a particular political candidate through PT-PAC may conflict with PTs' desire to support another candidate for other reasons. For instance, although a candidate may be a friend of physical therapy, he or she may support other social issues with which a PT does not agree. However, donations to a PAC are made with no strings attached. The donations are pooled and distributed in the best interest of PTs in general at both the state and federal levels.

Engaging in the political process to influence legislators is becoming increasingly important. Numbers speak volumes when lobbyists speak for PTs, and because the APTA is the organization that represents PTs in this country, PTs who are not members of the organization may have limited, if any, information on the issues and their impact on their practice. Consequently, these PTs may miss many opportunities to effect change that directly affects their practice of physical therapy. For example, if 300 PTs lived in a legislator's district and each one sought the legislator's support for an action important to the profession, the legislator might respond differently than if only a few PTs were heard from.

The comfort level of PTs in assuming responsibility for direct interactions with legislators varies widely. PTs who are not registered to vote or who do not exercise their right to vote may not be engaged enough in the political process even to identify the people who represent them, and contacting those representatives may be an intimating experience.

FURTHER THOUGHTS

Contemporary issues in physical therapy present many challenges to the profession and to individual PTs and PTAs. As they plan their professional development, individuals must identify the issues that affect their ability to fulfill their professional obligations to patients and determine the need for action from the professional organization that represents them. Individuals must be involved in the policy making of the APTA to proactively set the direction for physical therapy as well as to play a role in the achievement of its current goals.

QUESTIONS FOR REFLECTION

1. Although the 2020 vision statement calls for all PTs to have the DPT degree, accreditation requires only that the degree awarded at the postbaccalaureate level. What, if any, is the problem with this? Why have the requirements remained unchanged?
2. PTs with bachelor's degrees say that they were not offered opportunities for a transition master's degree as PT programs moved to the postbaccalaureate level, yet they are expected to seek clinical doctoral degrees. Why is there a greater urgency for all PTs to have the DPT degree?

3. The PTET provides information to academic programs that may be used to exempt students from course content in which they are competent. Does this seem to be a reasonable approach to determining who receives a t-DPT degree? Why or why not?

4. List the major challenges the profession faces in expanding its role in health, prevention, and wellness services? Also list the major challenges for individual PTs.

5. Should PTAs be awarded a bachelor's degree for their course of study? Why or why not?

6. What is the most important issue arising from the interdependent relationship of PTs and PTAs?

7. Do the benefits of autonomous, direct-access practice outweigh the risks for individual PTs?

8. You have decided to budget $500 next year for PAC donations. How do you decide which PAC to support when the APTA and two other organizations that promote causes important to you all seek your donation?

9. How would you prioritize the contemporary issues presented in this chapter for attention from APTA staff members?

10. Is the 2020 *Vision Statement* self-serving, or is it focused on the place of physical therapy in society? Explain your answer.

REFERENCES

1. American Physical Therapy Association. *APTA Vision Sentence and Vision Statement for Physical Therapy 2020* [HOD 06-00-24-35]. Retrieved November 11, 2003, from http://www.apta.org/About/aptamissiongoals/visionstatement

2. Threlkeld AJ, Jensen GM, Royeen CB. The clinical doctorate: A framework for analysis in physical therapist education. *Phys Ther* 1999;79:567-581.

3. Letters to the Editor. The DPT. *Phys Ther* 1999;79:978-990.

4. American Physical Therapy Association. *Transition doctor of physical therapy (DPT) degree.* Retrieved November 11, 2003, at http://www.apta.org/Education/transitiondpt/tdpt_faq

5. American Physical Therapy Association. *2002 PTA fact sheet.* Retrieved November 11, 2003, at http://www.apta.org/pdfs/accreditation/PTAFactSheet2002.pdf

6. American Physical Therapy Association. *Clinical specialization.* Retrieved November 11, 2003, at http://www.apta.org/Education/specialist/WhyCertify/OverviewSpecCert

7. American Physical Therapy Association. *Amended minimum eligibility requirements.* Retrieved November 11, 2003, at http://www.apta.org/Education/specialist/whycertify/OverviewSpecCert/MinEligRegsDetail#minimum%20el

8. American Physical Therapy Association. *Elements of the clinical specialization program.* Retrieved November 11, 2003, at http://www.apta.org/Education/specialist/whycertify/OverviewSpecCert/SpecCertOverviewDetail#Clinical Specialization

9. American Physical Therapy Association. *Employers' view of clinical specialists.* Retrieved November 11, 2003, at http://www.apta.org/Education/specialist/WhyCertify/Employers_View

10. American Physical Therapy Association. *Direct access.* Retrieved November 11, 2003, at http://www.apta.org/reimb/payer/diraccess

11. American Physical Therapy Association. *States that permit physical therapy treatment without referral.* Retrieved November 11, 2003, at http://www.apta.org/Documents/Public/GovtAffairs/directAccessLaws0803.pdf

12. American Physical Therapy Association. *Direct access to physical therapists' services.* Retrieved November 11, 2003, at http://www.apta.org/Govt_Affairs/state/directaccess/State2

13. American Physical Therapy Association. *A summary of direct access language in state physical therapy acts*. Retrieved November 11, 2003, at http://www.apta.org/pdfs/gov_affairs/directalaws

14. Taylor TK, Domholdt E. Legislative change to permit direct access to physical therapy services: A study of process and content issues. *Phys Ther* 1991;71:382-389.

15. Durant TL, Lord LJ, Domholdt E. Outpatient views on direct access to physical therapy in Indiana. *Phys Ther* 1989;69:850-858.

16. Domholdt E, Durchholz AG. Direct access use by experienced therapists in states with direct access. *Phys Ther* 1992;72:569-574.

17. American Physical Therapy Association. *Interactive guide to physical therapist practice with catalog of tests and measure* (version 1.0). Alexandria, Va: The Association; 2002.

18. Richardson JK. *Chance to grow*. Retrieved November 11, 2003, at http://www.apta.org/pt_magazine/jan98.html/pres.htm

19. Richardson JK. *Metamorphosis of RC 40-97 to RC 1-98*. Retrieved November 1, 2003, at http://www.apata.org/pt_magazine/May 98.html/pres.htm

20. Killen MB. Supportive personnel in physical therapy. *Phys Ther* 1967;47:483-490.

21. Watts NT. Task analysis and division of responsibility in physical therapy. *Phys Ther* 1971;51:23-35.

22. Figueroa-Soto I, Urmansky S, Hughes C et al. Uniqueness of physical therapy tasks and its relationship to complexity and delegation: A survey of Pennsylvania physical therapists. *J Allied Health* 1999;28:148-154.

23. Robinson AJ, DePalma MT, McCall M. Physical therapists' perceptions of the roles of the physical therapist assistant. *Phys Ther* 1994;74:571-582.

24. Robinson AJ, DePalma MT, McCall M. Physical therapist assistants' perceptions of the documented roles of the physical therapist assistant. *Phys Ther* 1995;75:1054-1066.

25. American Physical Therapy Association. *Evaluative criteria for accreditation of education programs for the preparation of physical therapist assistants*. Retrieved November 11, 2003, at http://www.apta.org/Education/accreditation/eval_criteria_menu

26. American Physical Therapy Association. *APTA physical therapist assistant employment survey: Fall 2001 executive summary*. Retrieved November 11, 2003, at http://www.apta.org/Research/survey_stat/pta_employ_nov01

27. American Physical Therapy Association. *Guide to physical therapist practice*. *Phys Ther* 1997;77:1163-1650.

28. American Physical Therapy Association. *What is PAC?* Retrieved November 11, 2003, at http://www.opensecrets.org/pacs/pacfaq.asp

29. US Federal Election Commission. *About the FEC*. Retrieved November 11, 2003, at http://www.fec.gov/about.html

30. American Physical Therapy Association. *Support PT-PAC*. Retrieved November 11, 2003, at http://www.apta.org//rt.cfm/Govt_Affairs/federal/ptpac/contributetoptpac

31. American Physical Therapy Association. *Successful election cycle for PT-PAC*. Retrieved November 11, 2003, at http://www.apta.org/pt_magazine/Feb99/policy_brief.html

32. American Physical Therapy Association. *PT-PAC*. Retrieved November 11, 2003, at http://www.apta.org/membership/involved/participate_governance/appointed_groups_info#ptpac

4

The Physical Therapist as Patient/Client Manager

The physical therapist integrates the five elements of patient/client management—examination, evaluation, diagnosis, prognosis, and intervention—in a manner designed to optimize outcomes.

– The Interactive Guide to Physical Therapist Practice with Catalog of Tests and Measures version 1.0 (2002)[1]

PATIENT/CLIENT MANAGEMENT

Although the term *patient/client management* is relatively new, this is probably the best established and most recognizable role of the physical therapist (PT). Yet patient/client management for the PT has changed over the years in five areas:
- Knowledge and skill used in the processes of evaluation and diagnosis, prognosis, and discharge planning
- Referral relationships with physicians
- Technological advances in the tools available for examination and intervention
- Interpersonal relationships with patients and clients
- Outcomes of care

EVALUATION AND DIAGNOSIS

Evaluation is the process of making clinical judgments, based on examination data, to create a problem list for each patient. Because this list may include problems that require referral of the patient to other professionals,[1] the PT first must establish which problems fall within the scope of practice of physical therapy, and for those, determine whether the problems require the skilled services of a PT. This decision-making process may also be considered clinical problem solving, diagnosing, or clinical reasoning. The end product of evaluation is a *diagnosis*, which is the term for problems that have been categorized into defined clusters, syndromes, or categories.[1]

Use of the Term Physical Therapy Diagnosis

Rose[2] clarified the issues surrounding use of the term *physical therapy diagnosis*. He suggested that using the term is important to distinguish the PT's findings from, and to complement, diagnoses made by other health care practitioners. Physical therapy diagnoses help identify the role of physical therapy and its scope of practice. Nevertheless, some have opposed the idea of PTs using the term *diagnosis,* expressing concerns about PTs' prerogative to diagnose in the first place and the extent of their involvement in the process. However, Rose[2] points out that, in physical therapy, Sahrmann[3] defined the term *diagnosis* as simply the primary dysfunction toward which the PT directs treatment, and this has helped dispel the fears of the medical community that PTs intend to diagnose disease, infringe on the practice of others, or perform clinical services outside their scope of expertise.

Rose[2] further explained that, by naming and classifying clusters of symptoms, signs, and demographic data (some obtained from similar patients who responded successfully to a specific treatment), the clinician increases the probability that the best results previously obtained will be replicated or surpassed. The diagnoses PTs select also help them share their results with other PTs. At the least, a diagnosis brings some psychological comfort to the PT and the patient; labeling the problem gives it a sense of reality and makes communication easier.

For the profession as a whole, physical therapy diagnosis achieves the following[2]:
- It eliminates the search for a common treatment for all patients, because diagnosis decreases the generalization of clinical problems.
- It provides an experiential basis, rather than hypothetical mechanisms, in which to ground physical therapy theory.
- It ensures the homogeneity of patients in comparison groups for research.

Diagnosis as Clinical Decision Making

Over the years a variety of models and approaches for general clinical decision making in physical therapy have been presented, in addition to specific frameworks for particular diagnostic groups. Steiner et al.[4] suggested a patient-centered clinical problem-solving process that incorporates the *International Classification of Functioning, Disability, and Health (ICF)* model devised by the World Health Organization (WHO).

Using the WHO model,[5] which serves as the common language for rehabilitation in almost 200 countries, Steiner et al.[4] created the rehabilitation problem-solving form (RPS-Form) (Figure 4-1). The form is helpful for discussing the process of clinical decision making that is consistent with other models used to guide PTs, such as the modified Nagi model[1] and the hypothesis-oriented algorithm for clinicians (HOAC) developed by Rothstein and Echternach,[6] which these authors updated to reflect terminology in the American Physical Therapy Association's *Interactive Guide to Physical Therapist Practice with Catalog of Tests and Measures*[1] and to include the prevention aspects of physical therapy.[7]

The biopsychosocial model of Steiner et al.[4] addresses health and disability at the biological (body function and structure), individual (activities), and social (participation) levels. These levels are the link between the interaction of a person's health condition (disease or disorder) and the personal and environmental factors that affect it. The RPS-Form allows the patient's point of view to be recorded, in his or her own words. The PT's point of view at each level of the model is documented, including the practitioner's hypotheses about the personal and environmental factors that may influence the problems identified either positively or negatively. Although designed for interdisciplinary rehabilitation, the RPS-Form may also be useful for PTs who are not part of such a team.

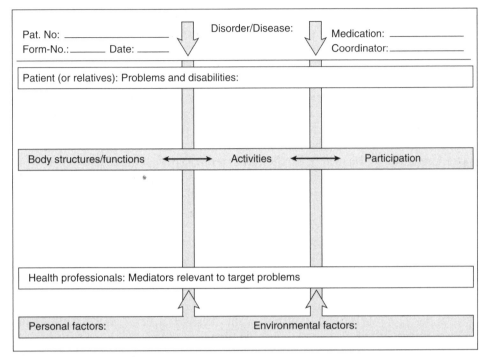

Figure 4-1. Rehabilitation problem-solving form (RPS-Form). The form is based on the World Health Organization's International Classification of Function, Disability, and Health (ICF) model. The form has three parts: (1) a header, in which basic information is recorded; (2) a section in which patients or relatives state their perception of the problem; and (3) a section in which health care professionals' analyses are presented. *(Courtesy Dr. Werner Steiner, Switzerland.)*

In Steiner's model[4] the more commonly held linear relationship (i.e., impairments lead to functional limitations, which lead to disability) is displaced. As Jette[8] points out, improvements in muscle strength (a reduction in an impairment outcome) assume that a commensurate reduction in disability (or improvement in patient functioning) will follow. PTs know that this is not necessarily true, because the relationship between force production and function is not linear; many complex factors influence this relationship. Use of the RPS-Form, instead of more traditional documentation formats, may help PTs make the shift away from a linear approach to problem solving.

PROGNOSIS

Prognosis is the determination of the predicted optimal level of improvement in function, the time needed to reach that level, and the levels of improvement that may be reached at various intervals during the course of physical therapy.[1] The prognosis is documented in the physical therapy plan of care, which includes the following:
- Specific short- and long-term goals for identified problems
- The duration and frequency of specific interventions selected to meet goals
- The expected outcome
- The optimal level of improvement expected

As the documentation of patient/client management, the plan of care reflects the result of the PT's evaluative process and the specific interventions to be used in an episode of care to accomplish specific goals and outcomes. Very little is known about physical therapy prognosis, but HOAC II[7] provides some suggestions for improving the goal-setting component of a traditional plan of care that address Jette's concerns about the link between impairments and functional limitations.[8]

The HOAC II model[7] specifies the types of goals as long term or short term. Long- and short-term goals represent the same kind of phenomenon (meaningful change for the patient); the only difference is the time required to achieve them. Defining goals in this way is an attempt to reduce confusion created by PTs who use short-term goals to reflect the impairments to be addressed so that long-term functional goals can be met. Because impairment changes, which are monitored through testing criteria, are not really goals, considering a change in impairment as the accomplishment of a goal is inappropriate. This viewpoint is supported by the fact that impairment changes may or may not result in improved function.

Patient function must therefore be addressed throughout a plan of care in short- and long-term goals that represent meaningful accomplishments. PTs can check whether a goal is meaningful by determining whether anyone, including the payer, would consider physical therapy worthwhile if only that goal were achieved.

As the PT's role in the prevention of illness gains strength and clarity, the practitioner faces another challenge in writing plans of care: goals related to the reduction or elimination of risk factors. PTs must be able to justify preventive interventions, often without supporting data. Without such data, unnecessary interventions may occur, or interventions may continue after they are no longer necessary.[7]

For the patient's current problems, PTs decide which interventions will achieve the short- and long-term goals. Jette and Jette[9] determined that this decision-making process is influenced by a variety of factors in addition to the patient's current health status. The PT's educational level, the payment source, the self-interests of the PT, and the size of the PT's caseload appear to be factors that contribute to treatment decisions.

Jette and Jette[9] also found that PTs' decisions about interventions were more homogeneous in cases involving patients with predictable diagnoses and prognoses for which the outcomes were generally agreed upon (e.g., individuals who had had knee surgery), than they were in cases involving patients for whom diagnosis was more difficult and the outcomes of treatment were less predictable (e.g., individuals with lumbar and cervical spine problems). Discharge planning presents similar challenges.

DISCHARGE PLANNING AND DISCONTINUANCE OF CARE

The *Interactive Guide to Physical Therapist Practice with Catalog of Tests and Measures,* published by the American Physical Therapy Association (APTA) and more commonly known simply as the *Guide,* makes a distinction between *discharge* from and *discontinuation* of physical therapy (Box 4-1).[1] Both terms are applied to the entire episode of physical therapy care, which the *Guide* defines as

> all physical therapy services that are provided by a PT, provided in an unbroken sequence, and related to the physical therapy interventions for a given condition or problem or related to a request from the patient/client, family, or other provider. The episode of care may occur exclusively under the care of only one PT in one practice, or it

Box 4-1   DISCHARGE AND DISCONTINUATION PROCESSES

Discharge

- *Discharge* is the process of ending physical therapy services provided during a single episode of care because the anticipated goals and expected outcomes of treatment have been achieved. *Note:* Discharge does not occur with a *transfer;* that is, when the patient is moved from one site to another site in the same setting or across settings during a single episode of care. Facility-specific or payer-specific documentation requirements may need to be met regarding the conclusion of physical therapy services as the patient moves between sites or across settings during the episode of care.
- Discharge is based on the physical therapist's analysis of the achievement of anticipated goals and expected outcomes. In consultation with appropriate individuals and in consideration of the goals and outcomes achieved, the physical therapist plans for discharge and provides for appropriate follow-up or referral.
- For patients/clients who require multiple episodes of care, periodic follow-up over the life span is needed to ensure the person's safe and effective adaptation to changes in physical status, care-givers, environment, or task demands.

Discontinuation

- *Discontinuation* is the process of ending physical therapy services provided during a single episode of care because of the following circumstances:
  1. The patient/client, caregiver, or legal guardian declines to continue intervention.
  2. The patient/client is unable to continue to progress toward anticipated goals and expected outcomes because of medical or psychosocial complications or because financial or insurance resources have been expended.
  3. The physical therapist determines that the patient/client will no longer benefit from physical therapy.
- When physical therapy services must be terminated before anticipated goals and expected outcomes have been achieved, the status of the patient/client and the rationale for discontinuation are documented.
- In consultation with appropriate individuals and in consideration of the anticipated goals and expected outcomes toward which therapy had been directed, the physical therapist plans for discontinuation and provides for appropriate follow-up or referral.

Modified from American Physical Therapy Association. *Interactive guide to physical therapist practice with Catalog of Tests and Measures.* Version 1.0. Alexandria, Va: The Association; 2002. This material is copyrighted, and any further reproduction or distribution is prohibited.

may include transfers among sites within or across settings or reclassification of the patient/client from one preferred practice pattern to another.[1-3]

For example, in an episode of physical therapy care, a patient who has undergone surgery for repair of a fractured femur may move from acute care to subacute or skilled nursing care to home care to outpatient physical therapy.

Discharge Planning

Discharge plans are completed at each transfer point in an episode of care. The requirements for these plans are established by the health care accreditation and licensing agencies for each type of institution and by governmental and private health care insurance regulations. Box 4-2, for example, presents a Medicare memorandum on discharge planning. The intent of these regulations is to contain costs, improve outcomes, and reduce the need for readmission to the hospital. Physical therapy practice acts may also address the PT's legal responsibility for discharge

---

Box 4-2 **Medicare Memorandum on Discharge Planning**

The Medicare conditions of participation (COP) for hospitals establish the following provisions.

Discharge Planning (42 CFR, §482.43 [b], 3 and 6)

Hospitals must have in effect a discharge planning process that applies to all patients, and the discharge planning evaluation must include an evaluation of the likelihood of a patient needing post-hospital services and of the availability of the services. The hospital must include the discharge planning evaluation in the patient's medical record for use in establishing an appropriate discharge plan, and the hospital must discuss the results of the evaluation with the patient or individual acting on his or her behalf. In addition, under *42 CFR, §482.43 (c)*, the patient and family members must be counseled to prepare them for post-hospital care.

Transfer or Referral (42 CFR, §482.43 [d], 5)

The hospital must transfer or refer patients, along with necessary medical information, to appropriate facilities, agencies, or outpatient services as needed for follow-up or ancillary care. Hospitals therefore should counsel beneficiaries discharged to receive home health services that their "primary" home health agency (i.e., the agency establishing the individual's plan of care) will provide all services. Hospitals should provide a list of home health agencies from which beneficiaries can choose; in addition, when referring the beneficiary to the chosen home health agency, the hospital should notify the agency and include any counseling notes, which should serve as a reminder to the agency also to notify the beneficiary that *all* services will be provided by the facility as the "primary" home health agency. Hospitals play a key role in making patients and their caregivers aware of Medicare home health coverage policies and in helping to ensure that those services are provided in the appropriate venue.

From Centers for Medicare and Medicaid Services. Program memorandum intermediaries, Department of Health and Human Services (DHHS), Centers for Medicare and Medicaid Services (CMS). Transmittal A-02-106, October 25, 2002. Retrieved November 9, 2003, at http://cms.hhs.gov/manuals/pm_trans/a02106.pdf

---

planning. Figure 4-2 shows a sample form PTs could use to ensure that these requirements are met.

The way in which PTs make discharge decisions is important. Jette, Grover, and Keck[10] studied occupational therapists and PTs in acute care settings to explore this decision-making process. They developed a model that reflects how therapists use their own experience to assess patient factors and arrive at an appropriate discharge plan, which is modified by health care regulations and consultation with others (Figure 4-3). It might be argued that PTs in any setting approach discharge planning in a similar manner.

In hospitals, nursing homes, and rehabilitation centers, discharge planning is usually a multidisciplinary process led by a social worker or case manager. Some negotiation among the health care professionals involved may be required to ensure that the patient goals of the individual providers coincide. For example, a patient may be medically stable but unable to function safely and independently enough to return home and negotiate flights of steps. The PT may feel that another two or three sessions would enable the patient to meet stair-climbing goals, but the rest of the team may recommend transfer to a skilled nursing home for more rehabilitation.

For patients in some of these settings, and for individuals receiving outpatient physical therapy treatment, the discharge decision may be made without input from all care providers. A patient may be discharged unexpectedly, surprising a PT whose plan of care is not complete, particularly if the discharge occurs while the PT is off duty. In some cases this may occur because the discharge plan, like the plan of care, is driven by reimbursement policies. For example, in acute care facilities, reimburse-

---

IT'S A NEW WORLD REHABILITATION CENTER

Patient Discharge Summary Information

Name of Patient: **Diagnosis:**

Date of Admission: **Date of Discharge:**   **Total # PT treatment sessions:**

Reason for discharge: _____ satisfactory goal achievement _____ patient declines
to continue care _____ patient unable to work towards goals due to (medical) (psychological)
(other) complications.

Current physiological/functional/participation status:

Goal achievement and reasons if goals were not achieved:

Discharge Plan

1. Home program (briefly describe):

2. Referrals for additional services (dates and names):

3. Recommendations for follow-up PT (dates and names):

4. Family and caregiver training (dates and names):

5. Equipment provided:

Plan discussed with:

_____

Physical Therapist   Date

Figure 4-2. Sample discharge planning form.

---

ment is driven by *diagnosis-related groups (DRGs)*. With this arrangement, a hospital receives a prospective payment for a particular diagnostic group regardless of how long patients in that DRG are in the hospital. Discharge earlier than the days allotted for a DRG means that the hospital may make money; discharge delayed beyond the DRG timetable may mean a loss of revenue for the hospital.

Prospective payment systems are used in other settings as well, meaning that the number of visits over a specific period of time may be predetermined or authorized for a particular diagnosis. PTs may have to negotiate with representatives of third-party payers to modify the payment limitations, or some third-party payers may limit the

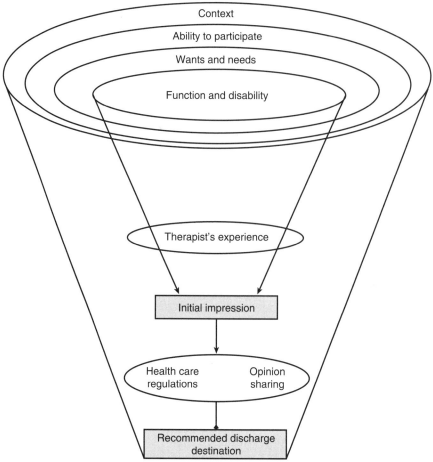

Figure 4-3. Dimensions of discharge decision making. (*Modified from Jette Du, Grover L, Keck CP. A qualitative study of clinical decision making in recommending discharge placement from the acute care setting.* Phys Ther *2003;83:224-236.*)

discharge destination to a particular type of setting. For instance, in an episode of care for a person with a total hip replacement, third-party intermediaries for Medicare may approve a 4-day postoperative clinical pathway to be implemented by all members of the health care team for that patient, then a transfer to a subacute care unit for 2 weeks, and then a transfer to home care three times a week for 1 month. Any deviation from this expectation requires that a PT, either alone or through the case manager, provide justification for postponing discharge at any transfer point in the episode of care.

Discontinuance of Care

In some cases the goals established in the plan of care cannot be met, either because the patient is unwilling or unable to participate or because the PT has decided the patient can no longer benefit from physical therapy; in this situation, services are considered to be discontinued, rather than the patient discharged. Detailed documentation of the reasons for discontinuance of care is important to ensure that patient abandonment is not an issue.

Bennett[11] defined *patient abandonment* as the unilateral severance of a professional relationship without reasonable notice when a necessity for continued care remains. The key to patient abandonment is failure of a PT to provide reasonable notice to a patient when the PT elects to end a professional relationship, regardless of the reason, and harm comes to the patient as a result. This legal concept has drawn attention to broader concerns about PT discharge decisions that are tied to restrictions on patients' financial resources (typically limited third-party payments for services). Bennett[11] suggested two critical courses of action for PTs:

1. Patients should be informed that limitations exist on the care that can be provided within the financial restrictions of their third-party payer.
2. Patients who need physical therapy services beyond their financial limits should be provided with options for continuing their care.

Examples of other means of continuing care include offering patients the option of paying for continued services with their own funds, assisting in appeals to third-party payers regarding the duration of care, or informing patients of other community-based programs through which care could be continued.[11]

OUTCOMES

According to the *Guide*, PTs ask themselves early in the patient/client management process, "What outcome is likely, given the diagnosis?"[1] After listing the likely outcomes for each diagnosis, they may reexamine the actual outcomes to determine whether the predicted outcomes are reasonable and then modify them as necessary. At the end of an episode of care, the PT informally reflects on, or formally analyzes through organizational review processes, the overall impact of the interventions on the patient's disorders, impairments, functional limitations, disabilities, health status, and satisfaction with care, as well as risk prevention, in terms of each likely outcome.[1] (Chapters 3 and 7 present more information on outcomes.)

The more PTs assume responsibility for practicing without referrals, the more accountable they will become for the outcomes of the care they provide. PTs who provide care as members of interdisciplinary teams face the challenge of determining the contribution of the physical therapy component to the outcome of the team effort.

CLINICAL DECISION MAKING

Regardless of which component of patient/client management PTs address at any point in time and which model they use in the process, they are making decisions at many levels. May[12] presents a model for this process that categorizes decisions along two continuums: from familiar to unfamiliar and from standardized to open (Figure 4-4).

May's model is useful for considering decisions in every component of patient/client management because, in the course of a day, all four types of decisions could be made in patient care. For instance, a pediatric PT may make the following kinds of decisions:

- *Standard familiar decisions:* The PT's knowledge and experience make these decisions almost automatic. For example, 85% of a PT's caseload may be made up of children with developmental delays. Patient/client management decisions for these patients are standard and familiar and become more so as the PT's knowledge of developmental delays and experience in working with these children increase.

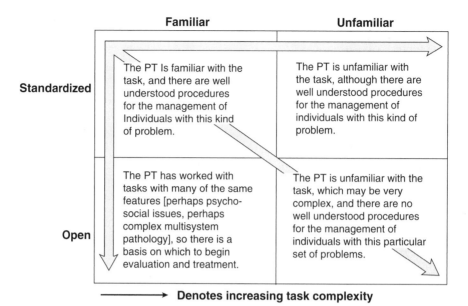

Figure 4-4. May's model of decision classification. *(From May BJ. Home health and rehabilitation. 2nd ed. Philadelphia: F.A. Davis: 1999.)*

- *Standard unfamiliar decisions:* The diagnosis and treatments for a condition are well known or at least supported by research but are not commonly encountered. For example, the same PT as above may be assigned a patient with torticollis; the PT is able to make decisions about the child's therapy but may feel less comfortable with or confident in patient/client management decisions for this new patient.
- *Open familiar decisions:* These are familiar decisions that involve some idiosyncratic element, such that further investigation or new strategies are required. For example, the pediatric PT may be assigned a new patient with developmental delays who also has visual and hearing impairments; the PT must therefore modify all the components of patient/client management to work effectively with the patient.
- *Open unfamiliar decisions:* These decisions involve confusing or conflicting information that requires longer and more careful consideration. For example, the parents of a child with developmental delays may request that the PT incorporate aromatherapy into the treatment sessions; otherwise they will take the child to another PT. Later the same day, the father of another patient tells the PT that he has lost his job and no longer has insurance to pay for the physical therapy services his child has been receiving regularly for over a year. In each case the PT must decide what action would be in the best interest of the patient.

In times of uncertainty, which typically arise from the instability of the larger environment in which PTs must practice, every decision may seem like an open unfamiliar decision. Changes in reimbursement policies, scientific evidence, and organizational structures contribute to the small percentage of open unfamiliar decisions PTs must face.[9]

A different type of model for clinical decision making is the hypothesis-oriented algorithm for clinicians mentioned previously.[7] Recently revised, HOAC II is a framework for science-based clinical practice that is grounded in the disablement terminology. It addresses the new challenges PTs face in goal setting to prevent problems and reduce risks for patients. In this two-part model, PTs are guided through clinical decisions for patients with existing problems and patients with possible future problems.

REFERRAL RELATIONSHIPS

PTs in the military and public health services routinely have practiced without referrals. However, through at least the 1960s, the general public typically had access to physical therapy services only through prescriptions written by physicians, who provided precise orders for each patient's plan of care. For example, the physician's orders detailed the output watts for ultrasound treatment, the duration of treatment, the number of repetitions and specific modes of exercise for particular muscle groups, and the water temperature for whirlpool treatments. For any modification, the PT had to contact the physician for a change in his or her orders.

This regimen is a far cry from current physical therapy practice in the United States. More than 30 states have passed legislation allowing the public direct access to PTs (and in 48 states PTs can perform initial examinations without a physician's referral).[13] More recently, at the federal level, legislation has been proposed that would allow direct access to physical therapy services for recipients of Medicare Part B benefits.[14] This is a key issue. Although direct access is widely permitted by law (a testament to legislatures' trust in PTs to care for those put directly in their charge), PTs routinely must provide evidence of physician's referrals in their claims for reimbursement.

However, the form of the required referral has changed. Most physicians now refer a patient for physical therapy without prescribing a detailed program; the referral simply reads, "Evaluate and treat." These changes have dramatically altered patient/client management by PTs, who have moved from the more technical role of implementing plans of care as instructed by prescription to total responsibility for the patient/client management process, from examination to outcomes.

As more PTs decide to practice without referral, determining the impact, if any, on patient/client management will be interesting. Many PTs already have a great deal of control over all elements of this process because they receive "evaluate and treat" referrals. The most likely changes will be an increased responsibility to refer a patient to a physician when the PT identifies problems beyond the scope of physical therapy practice and an increased responsibility for diagnosis and outcomes.

A shift may be seen in the physical therapy profession toward marketing directly to patients and also to physicians, who will continue to make referrals. Both physicians and patients will have more choices in directly selecting a PT, and in larger institutions they may comparison shop among PTs or physical therapy services. The skills of the PT in all elements of patient/client management may be examined much more closely by individuals who are self-referring than they are by patients who are referred and who assume that the referral is in their best interest. Establishing professional trust with the public may become more important than referrals in attracting potential patients directly and in seeking contracts with third-party payers, because both these groups will expect an accurate physical therapy diagnosis and outcomes that reflect the efficacy and efficiency of the care provided.

Reimbursement without a physician's referral has the potential to reduce health care costs because it requires fewer visits to the physician and less paperwork. However, opponents of direct access suggest that it may increase costs unless PTs are very good at determining the physical therapy diagnosis and, perhaps more important, the differential diagnoses, so that medical problems are not overlooked or incorrectly treated as movement problems, resulting in delayed medical diagnosis that may prove costly or even life threatening. The ability to perform a thorough systems screening as part of the history and examination is a critical skill, even when the physician has referred the patient primarily for confirmation of or the PT's contribution to the medical diagnosis. Without physician referral, the importance of the systems screening increases significantly.

Another recent issue in the business relationship between physicians and PTs stems from federal legislation controlling physician self-referral, or the Stark II law. The primary intent of the law is to protect Medicare beneficiaries from potential abuse of their benefits by physicians who refer patients for services and supplies in which physicians or their family members have a financial interest.[15] Self-referral also has the potential to limit opportunities for patients to seek the provider of their choice if they believe their only choice is the provider to whom the physician refers them. Physician employment of PTs has been on the decline over the years because of such measures limiting self-referral and because the number of PTs who are better prepared for and more interested in private practice has increased.

However, Stark II has the potential to reverse several of these trends because some of its provisions make exceptions to the definition of self-referral for ancillary services provided in-office under a physician's supervision. Many PTs are concerned about one of these exceptions, which may again increase the number of PTs employed by physicians and also, perhaps, the employment of non-PTs to deliver "physical therapy" in physicians' offices. The problem arises because the regulations are based on Current Procedural Terminology (CPT) billing codes (see Chapter 10) developed by the American Medical Association rather than professional or legal definitions of physical therapy.

The APTA has adopted a strategic plan for addressing the issue of physician-owned physical therapy services (POPTS).[16] The goals of this plan are to support statutory changes that would prevent POPTS, to identify the harmful effects of POPTS, to propose alternative opportunities for joint activities involving physicians and PTs, and to educate the public and PTs about the concerns inherent in POPTS.

TECHNOLOGICAL ADVANCES

Perhaps the most visible change in patient/client management has occurred in the tools available to PTs in tests, measurements, and interventions. Although considerable data can be collected without any equipment at all, and powerful physiological effects can be achieved when the PT's only tool is the hands, many electrical and mechanical devices have become available in patient/client management, and their use is limited only by the resources available to obtain them. A comparison of the equipment listed by Mary McMillan more than 70 years ago and that recommended in 1999 (Box 4-3) shows the advancements that have occurred in some areas—and also that some things have not changed (see Chapter 10).

Technological advances in surgical procedures, medical diagnostics, and pharmaceuticals also affect patient/client management in physical therapy. For example,

Box 4-3   COMPARISON OF PHYSICAL THERAPY EQUIPMENT LISTS: 1932 AND 1999

1932*	1999†
Wooden plinths	Mat tables
Several wooden stools of varying heights	Treatment tables
Small wooden blocks	Hi-low tables
Two wooden uprights for suspension of trapeze, large iron rings, Sayre head sling, pectoral stretching, paddle, and McKenzie apparatus	Isokinetic equipment
	Free-weight equipment
	Circuit training stations
	Rowing machine
Several pairs of dumbbells and Indian clubs	Pulley system
Large triple mirror	Therapeutic ball
Hydrotherapy plant for showers, douches, and sprays	Exercise bike
	Treadmill
Foot tubs	Parallel bars
High-frequency machine to deliver autocondensation	Balance beam
	Ballet bar
Three I-applicators with eight candescent lights	Stairs/ramp
	Balance equipment
Electric light cabinet	Tilt table
Portable high-frequency machine for diathermy, with accessories	Traction unit
	Portable mirror
Galvanic sinusoidal machine	Whirlpool
Galvanic controller with meter	Moist heat unit
Bristow faradic coil	Cold pack unit
Air-cooled ultraviolet	Fluidotherapy unit
Filing cabinet	Electrical stimulator unit
	Ultrasound machine
	Iontophoresis unit
	Executive desk and two side chairs
	Conference table and chairs
	File cabinet
	Personal computer and printer
	Carpeting, blinds, and artwork

*Modified from McMillan M. *Massage and therapeutic exercise* (3rd ed). Philadelphia: WB Saunders; 1932.
†Modified from Nosse LJ, Friberg DG, Kovacek PR. *Managerial and supervisory principles for physical therapists.* Baltimore: Williams & Wilkins; 1999.

arthroscopic techniques have dramatically reduced hospital stays and have led to a growth in the use of outpatient surgical procedures. New classes of drugs for treating arthritis and controlling neuromuscular disorders not only affect these patients' plans of care but also may reduce the need for physical therapy. Nevertheless, the more "high tech" health care becomes, the more "high touch" it needs to be.

INTERPERSONAL RELATIONSHIPS

In the 1977 Mary McMillan Lecture, Mary Clyde Singleton[17] reminded the physical therapy profession of the importance of its human side, seen in PTs' devotion to human welfare and in the need for PTs to be compassionate, loving, understanding, and conversant with the humanistic attributes of self and the relationship with others. This art of physical therapy, which is the profession's commitment to humane service, has not changed, but the challenges to the therapeutic relationship in which it must be achieved have. Some of these challenges, discussed elsewhere in the text, are as follow:

- The need to address a broader range of cultural issues
- Compliance with an ever-increasing number of laws, regulations, and ethical principles that guide physical therapy practice (discussed throughout the text)
- Third-party interpretation of regulations governing payment for services
- Increased access to information for both the PT and the patient
- Increased accountability and responsibility for care provided
- Less delegation of care to support personnel
- Employer productivity and caseload expectations
- Professional development of the PT
- Quality of evidence supporting PTs' decisions

In addition, the value placed on patients' participation in health care decisions has increased as PTs have moved away from the traditional paternalistic relationship between patients and care providers.

Using the Participation Method Assessment Instrument (PMAI), which they adapted from occupational therapy (Box 4-4), Baker et al.[18] explored the extent to which PTs encourage patients' participation in the planning of their care. Twenty-one identified opportunities are grouped in four components of the model. These are patient preparation, clarification of concerns, questions/statements, and actual goal setting. These possible interactions provide the opportunity for PTs to increase patient participation in plans of care by preparing the patient better with information the PT has gathered, clarifying the actual concerns that the patient may have, and providing opportunities for patients to ask questions.

The authors found that (1) PTs stated that including patients in goal setting was important and would improve outcomes and (2) patients believed that their inclusion was important. However, when the PTs' interactions with patients were analyzed, the researchers found that the PTs did not take full advantage of opportunities for patient participation (on average, 10 of the 21 opportunities were used). Suggested reasons for this lost potential for patient inclusion were impaired cognitive status of the patient, lack of time, and inadequate understanding or appreciation of the concept.

Although these concerns may be very important to PTs in the larger context of patient/client management, the key to successful outcomes still may be the PT's ability to establish a caring relationship with the patient. No matter what the technical ability or depth of knowledge, a PT who cannot establish a relationship in which the patient perceives caring may not be able to accomplish therapeutic goals. This premise was reinforced in a study of Swedish PTs who were asked to respond to a list of the potential factors in successful treatments (Box 4-5).[19] The results suggested that the patient's own strengths and the strength of the patient-therapist relationship are more important than treatment techniques in explaining why physical therapy works. Most of the participants in this study viewed physical therapy as a caring profession rather than an applied biomedical science.

Contemporary physical therapy faces no more demanding challenge than balancing the need to approach patient/client management scientifically, especially with the current emphasis on evidence-based practice (see Chapter 7), against the need to maintain powerful professional relationships with patients.

Box 4-4   USE OF THE PARTICIPATION METHOD ASSESSMENT INSTRUMENT (PMAI) IN PHYSICAL THERAPY

Patient Preparation

1. Physical therapy services are explained to the patient.
2. The patient is verbally prepared for initial and ongoing treatment.
3. Assessment purposes and procedures are presented to the patient, family, or significant others.
4. Assessment purposes and procedures are presented in a manner consistent with the level of understanding of the patient, family, or significant others.
5. Assessment findings are discussed with the patient, family, or significant others.
6. Assessment findings are discussed in a manner consistent with the level of understanding of the patient, family, or significant others.
7. The ways in which the individual is to participate in goal setting and treatment planning are discussed, unless such participation is contraindicated.
8. Patient is informed of the nature and potential outcomes of treatment.

Clarification of Concerns

9. The topic of exploration of concerns is introduced.
10. The patient's concerns are elicited.
11. Open-ended questions are used to gain more specific information about concerns the patient has expressed.
12. Clarification is used to gain more specific information about the patient's concerns.

Questions/Statements

13. The patient is asked to establish priority concerns.
14. The patient's major concerns are confirmed.

Goal Setting

15. The topic of exploration of goals is introduced.
16. The cooperative role of the patient in goal identification is explained.
17. The physical therapist collaborates with the patient, family, or significant others to establish goals.
18. The patient's stated concerns are incorporated into the exploration of goals.
19. Additional goals not identified by the patient but relevant to the person's rehabilitation are explored or explained.
20. The anticipated goals are presented to the patient, family, or significant others.
21. Goals are presented in a manner consistent with the level of understanding of the patient, family, or significant others.

Modified from Baker SM, Marshak HH, Rice GT, et al. Patient participation in physical therapy goal setting. *Phys Ther* 2001;81:1118-1126.

ETHICAL AND LEGAL ISSUES

Legal issues in patient/client management are addressed in state statutes, or practice acts, that regulate the physical therapy profession. PTs must be knowledgeable about the practice act in each state in which they intend to work, because the components of patient/client management and the factors that affect it may differ from one jurisdiction to another. Knowledge of state laws and legal ethical standards should be viewed as aspects of ongoing professional development (see Chapter 11). Professional ethics, however, are guided by professional documents common to all PTs as opposed to statutes that may be inconsistent from state to state.

Box 4-5   FACTORS IMPORTANT TO SUCCESSFUL PHYSICAL THERAPY TREATMENT

---

1. The physical therapist's treatment method is the most decisive factor in the patient's recovery.
2. A physical therapist should not become too involved with the patient's personal or social problems; these are the responsibility of other health care professionals.
3. Patient motivation is a vital component of successful therapy.
4. The interaction between the patient and therapist is crucial in physical therapy.
5. Physical therapy should promote the patient's health rather than emphasizing the diagnosis.
6. The physical therapist's knowledge and technique are what make physical therapy work.
7. The physical therapist should not simply treat a part of the body part, but rather should be interested in the whole person.
8. Physical therapy should be oriented toward the patient's resources rather than the person's problems.
9. The patient's own capacity for recovery is a major factor in the success of physical therapy.
10. Physical therapy is above all an aid to self-help; it works by eliciting the patient's own ability to change and improve.
11. The interaction between the physical therapist and patient that makes physical therapy successful begins during the first therapy session.
12. The physical therapist should place less emphasis on the patient's diagnosis and more emphasis on enhancing the individual's coping skills.
13. The interaction that occurs between the client and physical therapist has no bearing on a successful treatment outcome.
14. The patient's diagnosis should be the central focus of attention in physical therapy.
15. Many patients can be treated successfully without the physical therapist necessarily having a holistic view of the individual.

Modified from Stenmar L, Nordholm LA. Swedish physical therapists' beliefs on what makes therapy work. *Phys Ther* 1994;74(11):1034-1039.

Code of Ethics and Guide for Professional Conduct

As the term *patient/client management* might suggest, ethical issues related to this role of the PT focus on the relationship between the therapist and the patient, as well as the context in which these issues arise. For example, the APTA's *Guide for Professional Conduct*[20] (GPC) includes sections on confidentiality (GPC 2.3), trustworthiness, or fidelity, (GPC 2.1), respect for the individual's rights and dignity (GPC 1.1), and the autonomy of the patient (GPC 2.4). As stated in the GPC 2.1A, an appreciation of the vulnerability of the patient is fundamental to an understanding of the PT's responsibilities in patient/client management[20]:

> A physical therapist shall place the patient's/client's interests above those of the physical therapist. Working in the patient's/client's best interest requires knowledge of the patient's/client's needs from the patient's/client's perspective. Patients/clients often come to the physical therapist in a vulnerable state and normally will rely on the physical therapist's advice, which they perceive to be based on superior knowledge, skill, and experience. The trustworthy physical therapist acts to ameliorate the patient's/client's vulnerability, not to exploit it.

In short, patient/client management requires PTs to respect the patient's vulnerability, to step into the patient's shoes, and to act in the patient's best interest.

Autonomy

Autonomy refers to self-determination and is an important ethical principle in patient/client management. The principle of *patient autonomy* asserts that patients ought to have the right to make decisions about their health care. For example, the GPC states, "A PT shall respect the patient's/client's right to make decisions regarding the recommended plan of care, including consent, modification, or refusal" (GPC 2.4A).[20] The principles of confidentiality and informed consent are extensions of the basic principle of patient autonomy.

Informed Consent

Beauchamp and Childress[21] describe *informed consent* as having five elements: competence, disclosure, understanding, voluntariness, and consent. Although most PTs would agree that the PT has an obligation to obtain informed consent from the patient, some debate exists as to how this should occur and how the process should be described. In part, this debate stems from the differences between the PT's role and that of the physician. In many cases medical informed consent is obtained for a distinct medical or surgical procedure. In contrast, PTs may spend several hours each day with a patient; patient and therapists collaborate on a series of decisions that require continual disclosure and consent.

Some view informed consent as primarily a legal rather than an ethical concept, and statues covering informed consent for physical therapy may vary from state to state. For example, a Pennsylvania judge ruled in *Spence v. Todaro* that the concept of informed consent does not extend beyond surgical procedures.[22]

Scott[23] and Tygiel[24] presented opposing views of the PT's duty to obtain informed consent. Scott suggested that informed consent should always be obtained before spinal manipulation is performed and that administration of a written quiz related to the disclosed risks and benefits is necessary, to serve as documentation of the informed consent process.[23] Tygiel argued that manipulative procedures in physical therapy "do not present a high enough incidence of risk materializing for us to obtain informed consent with documentation."[24] A requirement to obtain written informed consent, he said, would expose the PT to unnecessary litigation for malpractice.

A review of APTA documents points up the uncertainty of the profession regarding appropriate procedures for obtaining informed consent. Although PTs quite clearly understand the need to obtain informed consent for patient/client management, the physical therapy profession is still in the process of reaching agreement on procedures for doing so. The following is a list of questions about informed consent in the physical therapy setting that remain unanswered:

- How should PTs ensure that they have obtained informed consent for patient/client management?
- What are the "material risks" of physical therapy patient/client management that must be disclosed to the patient?
- Is a significant enough risk associated with some physical therapy interventions to require written disclosure and consent?
- How should the profession determine what constitutes a risk? Would patients set a higher standard for disclosure and consent?
- Is the language of medical informed consent appropriate for physical therapy, or should different language be adopted that does not carry the legal baggage of this type of informed consent?
- If PTs abandon the language of informed consent, will some patients and PTs mistakenly believe that PTs have no obligation to obtain informed consent?

Regardless of the eventual answers to these questions, PTs have an ethical obligation to honor the right of patients to make decisions about their health care. True informed consent depends on a good relationship between the PT and the patient, characterized by continual communication. Managed care presents challenges to this relationship.

Managed Care and Fidelity

Recent changes in the health care delivery system, ushered in by managed care, illustrate how the organization of health care may affect the relationship between health care providers and patients. Morreim[25] describes the changes in managed care as posing a challenge to the age-old tenet of fidelity, which traditionally has meant that health care providers were bound to place the interests of their patients above other interests. However, in an attempt to put the brakes on escalating health care costs, managed care organizations have established financial incentives for providing fewer services. Morreim describes this as a "balancing act" in which health care providers must balance fidelity to the patient with accountability to society and financial self-interest. In this regard, Morreim[25] argues, conflict of interest is inherent to the managed care system.

The term *conflict of interest* may itself presume a pure and traditional concept of fidelity by subtly suggesting that multiple interests are always incompatible. However, as Beauchamp and Childress[21] observe, multiple loyalties may or may not be incompatible. Some ethicists use the term *divided loyalties*[21] or *double agency*[26] rather than *conflict of interest*. Regardless of the terminology, the managed care model aptly shows that the structure of the health care system has a significant impact on the relationship between the PT and the patient.

Peer-Reviewed Ethics Literature

A review of the ethics literature in physical therapy published from 1970 to 2000 found that the ethical aspects of patient/client management had been more extensively studied than the those aspects of the PT's other roles (i.e., consultant, educator, critical inquiry role, and administrator); 48.1% of peer-reviewed ethics articles were dedicated to patient/client management (Figure 4-5).[27] Informed consent, autonomy, confidentiality, relationship to patients, and ethical issues of health care organization were other, relatively frequent topics.

The APTA *Vision Statement* for the year 2020 looks to a future in which PTs will have privileges of autonomous practice and the public will have direct access to PT

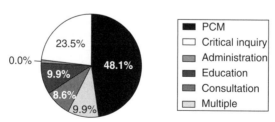

Figure 4-5. Roles of the physical therapist as described in peer-reviewed professional literature on ethics (1970-2000). (*Adapted from Swisher LL. A retrospective analysis of ethics knowledge in physical therapy; 1970-2000. Phys Ther 2002;82:692-706.*)

services in all settings. Since 1979 physical therapy leaders and ethicists[28-30] have warned that the increasing autonomy of physical therapy will bring more complex ethical dilemmas. With regard to the patient/client management role, PTs serving as autonomous practitioners in a direct access capacity undoubtedly will shoulder increased responsibility for screening for medical disease, referring patients to other health care practitioners, consultation with both individuals and organizations, and participating in policy formulation and patient advocacy. Given the lessons of managed care, these systemic changes in the PT's responsibilities may also cause changes in the PT-patient relationship. Attainment of the goals of the Vision 2020 statement will undoubtedly require further refinement of the ethical responsibilities implicit in the evolving patient/client management role.

FURTHER THOUGHTS

Patient/client management, the fundamental role of the PT, and the factors affecting it will continue to change. It therefore becomes essential for PTs to accomplish the management of each patient in the broader contexts in which physical therapy services are rendered.

CASE SCENARIOS

The following case scenarios address some of these issues.

Case Scenario 1

Libby Rubenstein has been seeking relief of her low back pain for over a year. She has been treated by four PTs in three different practices and continues to be unable to work at her job as a university English professor because of the pain. She is unable to drive her car without pain, and she feels that her relationship with her husband and two young children is suffering. She referred herself to you, the fifth PT, after exhausting her health insurance benefits for physical therapy.
- *Identify actions in the patient/client management process that may result in such a negative episode of care.*

Case Scenario 2

Juan Hernandez is a PT who routinely provides a physical therapy diagnosis in his reports to referring physicians. After receiving his first letter from Mr. Hernandez, Dr. Chan calls him to voice his shock that a PT had the nerve to make a diagnosis.
- *What would be an appropriate response to Dr. Chan?*

Case Scenario 3

A movement has arisen to revise the practice act in your state to make it illegal for PTs to *not* include patients in the planning of their physical therapy care.
- *Would you support this change? Why or why not?*
- *Assume that the revision is accepted. What five things do you think would be important to include in the rules accompanying the practice act?*

Case Scenario 4

Regional Orthopedic Services, a group practice of 12 orthopedic surgeons, has outsourced physical therapy services to a large rehabilitation corporation for the past 10 years. The time for renewal of that contract happened to coincide with implementation of the Stark II legislation, and the physicians have decided to hire their own PTs in-house rather than renewing the contract. An employment recruiter has called you to determine your interest in being one of the first of 10 PTs the group wants to hire to provide in-house physical therapy.

- *What questions do you have for the recruiter?*
- *What will be a key point in your decision about this opportunity?*

REFERENCES

1. American Physical Therapy Association. *Interactive guide to physical therapist practice with catalog of tests and measures* (version 1.0). Alexandria, Va: The Association; 2002.
2. Rose SD. Physical therapy diagnosis: Role and function. *Phys Ther* 1989;69:535-538.
3. Sahrman SA. Diagnosis by the physical therapist—a prerequisite for treatment. A special communication. *Phys Ther* 1988; 68(11):1703-1706.
4. Steiner WA, Ryser L, Huber E, et al. Use of the ICF model as a clinical problem-solving tool in physical therapy and rehabilitation medicine. *Phys Ther* 2002;82:1098-1107.
5. World Health Organization. *International classification of functioning, disability, and health.* Retrieved November 9, 2003, at http://www.who.int/icf/icftemplate.cfm
6. Rothstein JM, Echternach JL. Hypothesis-oriented algorithm for clinicians: A method for evaluation and treatment planning. *Phys Ther* 1986;66:1388-1394.
7. Rothstein JM, Echternach JL, Riddle DL. The hypothesis-oriented algorithm for clinicians II (HOAC II): A guide for patient management. *Phys Ther* 2003;83:455-470.
8. Jette AM. Outcomes research: Shifting the dominant research paradigm in physical therapy. *Phys Ther* 1995;75:965-971.
9. Jette DU, Jette AM. Professional uncertainty and treatment choices by physical therapists. *Arch Phys Med Rehab* 1997:78:1346-1351.
10. Jette DU, Grover L, Keck CP. A qualitative study of clinical decision making in recommending discharge placement from the acute care setting. *Phys Ther* 2003;83:224-236.
11. Bennett JJ. APTA examines patient abandonment. *PT Magazine* 1999;7:24-28.
12. May BJ. Twenty-eighth Mary McMillan Lecture: On decision making. *Phys Ther* 1996;76: 1232-1241.
13. American Physical Therapy Association. *A summary of direct access language in state physical therapy practice acts.* Retrieved November 9, 2003, at http://www.apta.org/Documents/Public/GovtAffairs/directAccessLaws0803.pdf
14. Massey BF Jr. 2002 APTA presidential address: What's all the fuss about direct access? *Phys Ther* 2002;82:1120-1123.
15. American Physical Therapy Association. *HCFA issues Stark II final regulations.* Accessed November 9, 2003, at http://www.apta.org/Govt Affairs/regulatory/fraud abuse/PhysSelfReferral starkII/starkIIFinal.
16. American Physical Therapy Association. Strategic plan addressing POPTS is adopted. *PT Bulletin Online.* Retrieved November 14, 2003, at http://www.apta.org/bulletin?&id[1]=46699#51978
17. Singleton MC. The Twelfth Mary McMillan Lecture: Do we dare to remember? *Phys Ther* 1977;7: 1264-1270.
18. Baker SM, Marshak HH, Rice GT, et al. Patient participation in physical therapy goal setting. *Phys Ther* 2001;81:1118-1126.

19. Stenmar L, Nordholm LA. Swedish physical therapists' beliefs on what makes therapy work. *Phys Ther* 1994;74:43-49.

20. American Physical Therapy Association. *APTA guide for professional conduct.* Retrieved October 21, 2004, at http://www.apta.org/AM/Template.cfm?

21. Beauchamp TL, Childress JF. *Principles of biomedical ethics* (ed 4). New York: Oxford University Press; 1994.

22. Scott R. Professional ethics: A guide for rehabilitation professionals. St Louis: Mosby; 1998.

23. Scott RW. Spinal manipulation and patient informed consent in orthopaedic physical therapy. *Phys Ther Orthop Pract* 2001;13:9-11.

24. Tygiel PP. Letter to the editor. *Orthop Pract* 2002;14:24-28.

25. Morreim EH. *Balancing act: The new medical ethics of medicine's new economics.* Washington, DC: Georgetown University Press; 1995.

26. Bruckner J. Physical therapists as double agents: Ethical dilemmas of divided loyalties. *Phys Ther* 1987;67:383-387.

27. Swisher LL. A retrospective analysis of ethics knowledge in physical therapy: 1970-2000. *Phys Ther* 2002;82:692-706.

28. Purtilo RB. Understanding ethical issues: The physical therapist as ethicist. *Phys Ther* 1974;54:239-242.

29. Magistro CM. Clinical decision-making in physical therapy: A practitioner's perspective. *Phys Ther* 1989;69:525-534.

30. Guccione AA. Ethical issues in physical therapy practice: A survey of physical therapists in New England. *Phys Ther* 1980;60:1264-1272.

The Physical Therapist as Consultant

5

"Consultation is the rendering of professional or expert opinion or advice by a physical therapist. The consulting physical therapist applies highly specialized knowledge and skills to identify problems, recommend solutions, or produce a specified outcome or product in a given amount of time on behalf of a patient/client."

– The Interactive Guide to Physical Therapist Practice with Catalog of Tests and Measures version 1.0 (2002)[1]

CONSULTATION IN BUSINESS

Definitive information about consultants is generally difficult to obtain, perhaps because consultants are by nature entrepreneurial, and the business is competitive. Even so, consultants long have been a mainstay of traditional businesses, helping their clients to solve work-related problems and assisting in decision making. More recently, consultants have emerged outside this primary arena, and the title now is applied to a wide range of service providers, from wedding planners to personal trainers.

Consultation has assumed this broader perspective because of the modern information explosion and a fluctuating marketplace, circumstances that have led more organizations and individuals to seek consultants for guidance, answers to questions, second opinions, and training. Consultants are also hired to serve as sounding boards for new ideas and strategies[2] and to provide expert advice for specific purposes.

The term *consultant* has become widely used in a variety of settings. The purposes of this chapter are to provide a clear picture of consultation in physical therapy, identify opportunities for physical therapy consultation, and consider the qualities of consultants.

PHYSICAL THERAPY CONSULTATION

Consultation is the practice of providing advice for a fee. This is a two-way interaction, a process in which a person or an organization seeks help, which the consultant provides.[3] The ultimate outcome of the process is a change in the way the person functions or an organization operates.[4] The person or organization seeking help is the *client*, who may also be known as the *customer, patient,* or *advisee*.[5] Regardless of the label applied to the interaction (advising, coaching, counseling, consulting), this helping process is a key function of all professionals, including physical therapists.

Given the nature of their work, most physical therapists (PTs) are familiar with the process of consultation. The patient/client management role of the PT is a form of consultation, because patient care is a process of giving and receiving help. By developing and implementing plans of care, PTs learn how to establish helping relationships with patients and ways to offer advice. These helping skills can easily be transferred to other consultation opportunities.

The power of the advice given depends on two factors: (1) how much the consultant helps clients use their own knowledge, experience, and expertise to arrive at a decision or solve a problem, and (2) how much the client participates in the proposed course of action.[5] In some consultation arrangements, the consultant provides an expert opinion that the client is expected to follow; in others the consultant draws upon the client's knowledge and expertise to help make the decision. More often, the consultation relationship falls somewhere in between. For instance, a faculty advisor often provides expert opinion while guiding students in making their own decisions about their careers. In the same way, PTs make every effort to move away from the paternalistic model of "doing for the patient"; instead, they try to use the active participation model, involving patients in decisions about their rehabilitation.

Maister, Green, and Galford[6] proposed four levels of consultation that define the consultant/client relationship. Box 5-1 presents examples of ways PTs might engage in consultation at each level.

Fuller[7] suggested another framework that consultants could use to clarify their responsibilities. This model identifies types of consultation in terms of client demands for the following continuum of services:

- Specialized services
- Administrative skills
- Problem solving
- Investigative studies
- Assessments
- Advice

Because some blurring of roles occurs in a consulting continuum between consultants at the specialized service-provider end and others at the advice-giving end, Fuller defined the consultant/client relationship as a blend of service and advice, with some specialized information added.[7] Often the precise boundary between the advising and the service-providing processes is vague, especially if the individual who gave the advice is then asked by the client to implement it.[5] This is often the case in physical therapy. For example, physical therapy consultants may help a business determine the physical therapy services it should have, and the PTs may then provide the services identified as the answer to the client's needs.

Physical therapy consultants are hired to meet a range of client needs. McGonagle and Vella[8] and Cohen[9] have identified broad categories of client needs that can be applied to physical therapy consultation (Table 5-1). Clearly, opportunities abound for PTs who seek helping relationships beyond patient/client management.

Box 5-1   EXAMPLES OF CONSULTATION SERVICES PROVIDED BY PHYSICAL THERAPISTS

Level 1: Service-Based Consultation

- A physical therapist (PT) consultant contracts to provide direct patient care services for a rural hospital on a temporary basis.
- A PT consultant contracts to develop a new specialty service for individuals with lung disease that developed secondary to occupational exposure.

Level 2: Needs-Based Consultation

- A physical therapy practice has a problem with a very high percentage of reimbursement denials from a particular third-party payer. The group hires a PT consultant to develop and implement a training program for the rehabilitation team that will provide guidelines for reimbursement and for effective documentation that supports charges for services.
- A physical therapy practice, overwhelmed by the process of complying with the rules and requirements of the Health Insurance Portability and Accountability Act (HIPAA), hires a PT consultant to develop procedures that will ensure that the practice is in compliance.

Level 3: Relationship-Based Consultation

- A PT consultant is hired by a newly formed physical therapy group to help develop its services from the ground up: mission statement, budgeting, policies and procedures, hiring criteria, and marketing strategies.
- A PT consultant is hired by the same group a year later to help determine whether the practice should expand into new markets.

Level 4: Trust-Based Consultation

- A physical therapist engages a consultant. They meet at least four times a year to brainstorm ideas for the physical therapist's practice and professional development.

Modified from Maister DH, Green CH, Galford RM. *The trusted advisor.* New York: Free Press; 2000.

Consulting PTs must also decide the type of clients with whom they want to work—physical therapy peers, others, or both. Few professionals set out to become consultants, and the transition to consultation as a sole source of income is often subtle and gradual.[10] A typical starting point for PTs would be the service-providing end of consultation, with perhaps some problem-solving work included. A physical therapy consultant's first clients often are other PTs because both consultant and client are comfortable with the jargon, and they have a professional camaraderie.

The initial consultation efforts often are opportunities PTs take in addition to their full-time employment. Eventually PTs may realize that their primary source of income has become consultation, at which point they disengage from full-time employment and identify themselves more as consultants than PTs. As the full-time consulting business grows, the level of consultation often changes; also, the PT consultant's client base may broaden to include other health care professionals or different types of health care and community organizations. Some PT consultants develop skills in organizational process, team building, or other consulting skills that do not require physical therapy expertise.

Generalist physical therapy consultants address a broad range of problems in physical therapy, but many consultants narrow their spectrum of expertise, for example, serving as physical therapy education consultants, physical therapy private practice development consultants, or physical therapy sports medicine consultants. Figure 5-1 presents a quick self-test to help PTs determine where their interests might lie in the complex world of consulting.

Table 5-1 | **Client Needs Met by Physical Therapy Consultants**

Circumstance	Consultant's Roles
Inadequate human resources	Make up for a shortage of a particular expertise among existing personnel
	Serve as an alternative when hiring restrictions are in place
	Help to manage a sudden increase in expectations or demand
	Provide services when time limits prevent existing personnel from completing the work at hand
	Work on a new project that does not warrant the hiring of full-time personnel
Objective point of view	Provide guidance or insight on a particular patient or management problem
	Present new ideas for revitalizing the practice
	Devise fresh approaches for overcoming barriers to successful treatment outcomes
Periods of change	Serve as a catalyst to help generate change in a health care organization
	Lend credibility to a change already determined to be necessary
	Provide seminars for or coaching of personnel to provide information and new skills to improve clinical practice
	Provide rapid access to latest technology and its application
	Serve as an independent mediator to resolve differences when two health care organizations merge
Business management	Improve referrals to the physical therapy service
	Research sources of capital funding to initiate a physical therapy practice
	Improve an organization's efficiency and scope of practice
	Ensure compliance with regulatory and accreditation demands or third-party payer rules for reimbursement
	Help with a complete turnaround in a practice resulting from a change in mission or organizational structure so that the practice remains competitive as health care changes occur

Modified from McGonagle J, Vella CM. How to use a consultant in your company: A managers' and executives' guide. New York: John Wiley & Sons; 2001; and Cohen W. How to make it big as a consultant (3rd ed). New York: Amacom; 2001.

The farther to the right the marks fall on each continuum in Figure 5-1, the more the PT becomes a true consultant. True consultation typically involves a one-time, short-term contract through which the consultant is hired for a specific task and released when the task is done. Consultants usually have more than one client at a time, or, at the least, are developing proposals for potential new clients while engaged with one client. Individuals typically are considered *professional consultants* when consultation is their only source of income.[7]

Consulting requires skills beyond the consultant's ability to convey expert knowledge and advice. For example, a number of skills are needed for the practical business aspects of consulting. A major component of a consultant's success is the ability to use entrepreneurial and business skills to build up and sustain a client list. Consultants must develop skills in identifying potential clients, marketing their

Place mark on each line indicating where you stand as a consultant

Moonlight	Consult as primary income
Generalist	Specialist
Provide advice to be taken	Lead client to own decision
Service only	Advice only

Figure 5-1. This quick self-test can help PTs determine where their interests might lie in physical therapy consulting. (Modified from Fuller GW. *Getting the most out of your consultant: A guide to selection through implementation.* Boca Raton, Fla: CRC Press; 2000.)

services, determining their effectiveness, and attending to the ethical aspects of consultation. Many self-help texts are available that address the business of consulting, and PTs should make use of them before deciding whether to rely on consulting as their only source of income.

BUILDING A CONSULTING BUSINESS

Consulting Fees

Consultants must be prepared to pay themselves and have money left for developing and managing the business. Although the value of the consultation ultimately is determined by the client, fees are determined by many factors. On the client's side, these factors include the type of business or industry, its size and location, the demand for consultants by such businesses, and the client's history of consultant use. On the consultant's side, factors include the individual's level of expertise, degree of experience, and professional standing. This supply-and-demand situation creates a wide price range for consultation. Competition also drives fees. For example, consultants who are moonlighting may accept projects for much lower fees because they have other income. Large organizations in metropolitan cities, which have more consultants from which to choose, may encourage bidding for projects.

The real question is how to determine how much clients should be charged. A billable daily fee can be arrived at in two ways.[11] First, the consultant can determine a fee with an income goal in mind. With this method, the consultant calculates the amount needed to cover living and business expenses for 1 year, determines the number of billable days in a year, and uses this information to arrive at a per-hour fee. The second method is to match the fees charged by other physical therapy consultants. Obtaining this information may be difficult because other professionals, wanting to keep a competitive edge, may be reluctant to share their fee schedules. Consultants often do their best to guess the amount they believe the client is willing to pay, present this as the fee, and hope the client agrees. In reality, consultants use both of these fee determination methods.

If clients think that the consultant's offer meets their needs, they most likely will pay the fee without questioning it. Starting high, therefore, is easier than increasing fees at a later time.[12] Box 5-2 presents the two methods of setting fees.

Box 5-2   ESTABLISHING CONSULTING FEES

Method 1

1. Calculate the amount you need to cover living and business expenses for 1 year.
2. Calculate the number of billable days in a year:
   - With 2 weeks of vacation, holidays, and weekends, a year has about 245 billable days.
   - Subtract 2 or 3 days per week for marketing activities, networking, handling the administrative aspects of the business, writing proposals, and engaging in professional development.
   - Typically 120 days per year are available for billable work (this number is affected by the scheduling of available days when clients are available; for example, a client may find it difficult to engage a consultant around the holidays in December. Consider the following example of estimated expenses and income for 1 year:

Salary	$50,000
Taxes	$20,000
Retirement	$7,500
Insurance	$6,000
Overhead business expenses	$25,200
Profit	$10,000
Total	$118,700

3. For this example, if you plan 80 billable days per year, your daily consulting fee would be about $1,500 a day.

Method 2

1. Determine the fee potential clients are willing to pay (e.g., find out the fee paid to other consultants in the area).
2. Determine your living and business expenses.
3. Calculate the number of consulting days per year you need to break even. For example, let's say the current daily fee for PT consultants in your area is $750, and your annual income goal is $118,700:

$$\$118,700 \div 750 = 158.26$$

You will need to work about 159 billable days per year to meet your income goal.

Many organizations and government agencies insist on a fixed price for projects, which often is determined through a request for proposal (RFP) process. The organization announces an RFP with a particular goal or product in mind. Several consultants submit proposals, including a fixed bid, and the organization selects the best proposal for the best price. This approach to setting a fee is riskier than the billable day approach, which allows consultants to renegotiate for more time as a project progresses or is modified. With a fixed-price project, the consultant assumes the risk of the total cost of the project, including the risk of actual costs exceeding the negotiated price.

At the service-providing end of the consultation spectrum, percentage fee arrangements may be used when the financial outcome of the project is clearly measurable and the consultant agrees to a percentage of profits.[12] For instance, a physical therapy consultant hired to reduce denials of reimbursement claims may base the fee on the percentage increase in dollars paid for claims submitted over the next 3 years.

Regardless of the method used, the consultant must determine a consistent pricing structure that applies to all clients for the same work. Prices may vary if some aspect of the work is different (e.g., on-site versus home-based consultation) or if the client is a nonprofit organization and the consultant chooses to give a discount. If the fee structure changes, the consultant, to avoid a tarnished image, must be clear about the reason for the change.

The Consulting Process

Parallels can be drawn between the patient/client management process in physical therapy and the true consulting process as described by Lippitt and Lippitt[3] (Figure 5-2). Like PTs, consultants identify problems, consider alternatives, select and implement the best solution, and evaluate the solution's effectiveness.

As entrepreneurs, consultants must market their services and seek out potential clients. As with any entrepreneurial business, as the consultant's reputation grows, potential clients may self-refer, or former clients may recommend new ones. The consultant/client relationship begins with acceptance of a proposal, which may be developed in response to an RFP or as a result of a preliminary meeting with a potential client. A strong consulting proposal hinges on a thorough knowledge of the client and the client's needs. The proposal should include the following sections, which are based on an outline by Hoyt[13]:

1. *Purpose of the proposal [or an objective]:* A brief statement, couched in general terms, of what the client wants.
2. *Solution or action steps:* Presented perhaps as a bulleted list or a table, this section specifies the sequential actions to be taken, including dates for submission of periodic progress reports. The steps may include information and data gathering, design, content to be included, materials needed, and the implementation strategy.

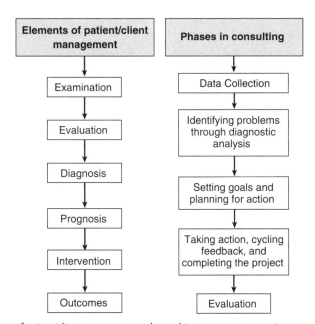

Figure 5-2. Comparison of patient/client management and consulting processes. *(From the American Physical Therapy Association. Interactive guide to physical therapist practice with catalog of tests and measures, version 1.0. Alexandria, Va: The Association; 2002 [this material is copyrighted, and any further reproduction or distribution is prohibited]; and Lippitt G, Lippitt R. The consulting process in action (2nd ed). San Francisco: Jossey-Bass; 1986.)*

3. *Anticipated benefits:* The improvements the client can expect as a result of the consultation.
4. *Evaluation:* A plan for measuring the effectiveness of the consultation.

At any level of consultation, consultants must do their homework to develop proposals that are attractive to clients. The consultant must learn everything possible about a client and about the factors that influence the client's decision making and goals so as to identify clearly problems and possible solutions.

The Skills of a Good Consultant

Consultation demands skills beyond good advice, technical capabilities, and entrepreneurial talent. Other required skills include the ability to get along well with others, the ability to diagnose problems and find solutions, the ability to communicate, and the ability to work under pressure.[9] Some personal qualities and attitudes are also critical. Consultants must be adventuresome, willing to accept risk, and determined to find answers to problems.[13] PTs develop many of these skills in patient care and others as managers of patient care services and can transfer these capabilities to the consultant's role. As in any other career choice, PTs who decide to pursue consulting should take the time to reflect on their strengths and weaknesses and prepare accordingly. Figure 5-3 presents a list of questions[11] that can be helpful to PTs considering this decision.

Even when all the appropriate skills are in place, the key to success as a consultant is the ability to build a trusting relationship with the client.

Respond to each item using a 1–4 scale.

1 = definitely true; 2 = possibly true; 3 = unlikely; 4 = definitely false

1. I am willing to work sixty to eighty hours a week to achieve success.	1	2	3	4
2. I love risk; I thrive on risk.	1	2	3	4
3. I have a thick skin.	1	2	3	4
4. I am good at understanding and interpreting the big picture.	1	2	3	4
5. I pay attention to details.	1	2	3	4
6. I am an excellent communicator.	1	2	3	4
7. I am a good writer.	1	2	3	4
8. I like to sell myself.	1	2	3	4
9. I can balance logic with intuition and the big picture with details.	1	2	3	4
10. I know my limitations.	1	2	3	4
11. I can say "no" easily.	1	2	3	4
12. I am compulsively self-disciplined.	1	2	3	4
13. I am comfortable speaking with people in all disciplines and at all levels of an organization.	1	2	3	4

Figure 5-3. This short quiz can help PTs decide whether consulting might be a prospect for them. *(From Biech E. The business of consulting: The basics and beyond. San Francisco: Jossey-Bass/Pfeiffer; 1999.)*

Trust in the Consultant/Client Relationship

Consultants must be able to give their clients objective, independent advice that is unaffected by the client's own biases, fears, and blind spots. However, consultants must also be alert to their own biases, fears, and self-interests and take steps to guard against them. They can guard against these personal foibles by attending to their obligations to their clients: loyalty and care. As in patient/client management, consultants must place clients' interests above their own and look after those interests carefully.[5]

Clients often have mixed feelings about consultants that affect the consultant-client interaction. On one hand, clients may respect consultants for their unique skills or ability to resolve problems. On the other hand, clients may view consultants with skepticism because of the perception that they profit from the weaknesses of others. The presence of a consultant may suggest that the client has weaknesses and is unprepared to deal independently with the issues at hand. A client's employees may see the hiring of a consultant as a red flag, signaling impending changes that may be unwelcome.[7]

Establishing trust is critical to overcoming these hurdles. A consultant who puts the client's interests first and is sensitive and careful in interactions with the client and others affected greatly improve the chances of success. Trust is earned through direct experience in a highly personal, emotional, and dynamic two-way relationship that involves risk on both sides.[6]

Because the client must feel free to accept or reject the consultant's advice, the consultant is responsible for organizing and directing the consultation process toward the desired end of solving a problem. Trusting and being trusted are critical to the delicate balance that must be achieved if a consultant is to bring the client to decisions that are in the client's best interests without appearing to be righteous or self-serving. To begin establishing trust, the consultant must honestly determine whether the consultation will contribute a worthwhile component in an effective manner to the problem or objective.[6]

A consultant must be sensitive to the position of clients, who put themselves on the line when retaining consultants. Clients' reputations are at stake, because they will be evaluated on the results of the consultation. Clients need to feel confident that the consultant will do a thorough, professional job.

In the end, consulting is primarily a relationship business. Without that relationship, the consultant's specialized knowledge and experience are of no value. Also, the consultant's success depends heavily on the quality of the relationship that develops as the process moves toward the desired goal. The legal and ethical ramifications of this trust relationship are paramount.

ETHICAL AND LEGAL ISSUES IN CONSULTATION

The consultant role of the PT raises a number of legal and ethical issues, many of them related to the type and setting of the consultation. This section addresses the legal status of employment; relevant portions of the *Code of Ethics* and the *Guide for Professional Conduct*, both published by the American Physical Therapy Association (APTA); institutional review boards for the protection of the rights of research subjects; and the differences between patients and research subjects.

Legal Status of Employment

Consultants act *with* a system rather than as an integral part of it. However, the substance of the relationship, rather than the label it is given, determines the consultant's legal employment status. No legal status exists for a *consultant* per se. Labor laws distinguish between *employees* and *self-employed contractors*. Box 5-3 presents a comparison of the two groups of workers.[2] The consultant is an independent contractor more than an employee. In an independent contractor agreement, a client hires an expert to perform a certain task, relinquishes control over the way the task is accomplished, and is relieved of certain legal responsibilities of employers.[8]

However, the farther the consultant's task is from the center of the service–advice continuum, the less the consultant is like an independent contractor. For example, at the advice end, the specific task or service to be delivered may be less clear; at the service end, the client may have significant control over patient assignments or scheduling.

If the answer to each of the following six questions is "yes," the individual's employment status is likely to be that of consultant[8]:

1. Are you generally free to seek out many business opportunities and to work for more than one client at a time?
2. Are you paid a flat, negotiated fee for your work?
3. Do you provide your own resources to get the job done?

Box **5-3**   COMPARISON OF EMPLOYEE AND SELF-EMPLOYED CONTRACTOR STATUS

Employee Status	Self-Employed Contractor Status
• The intention of the employer and employee is to form an employment relationship, which is reflected in ally written agreement or correspondence and/or by the behavior of the parties involved. • The employer or an agent controls the hours worked. • The employer or an agent has the power to hire and fire. • The employer incurs the profit or loss from the enterprise. • The employer deducts ACC premiums and pays taxes on behalf of the employee. • The employer supplies the materials for the work. • The employer owns or leases the equipment needed for the work. • The employee is bound to one employer at a time and is expected not to compete with the employer or to offer his or her skills to the employer's competitors.	• The intention of the parties to the contract is not to form an employment relationship, and the actual nature of the relationship reflects this. • The contractor controls how and when the job is done. • Payment is made in a lump sum at the end of a job or in installments as the job progresses. • The contractor can choose who does the job and can hire other people without approval from the other party. • The contractor pays any taxes and ACC and insurance premiums directly. • The contractor may make a profit or suffer a loss directly. • The contractor supplies the equipment and materials for the job. • The contractor is free to accept similar work from a number of sources at the same time.

Modified from U.S. Internal Revenue Service. *Independent contractor or employee.* Retrieved November 21, 2004, at http://www.irs.gov/pub/irs.pdf/p1779.pdf; and New Zealand Department of Labour. *Who is an employee and who is not?* Retrieved November 9, 2003 at http://www.ers.dol.govt.nz/relationships/employee.html

    4.   Are you at risk for suffering a loss if your estimated expenses are exceeded?

    5.   Is there *no* expectation that the work will continue indefinitely?

    6.   Is the work you are doing *not* considered a routine part of the organization?

Contract Law

Because the legal definition of consulting is unclear, a consulting agreement or contract must clearly delineate the factors that establish, maintain, and terminate the consultant-client relationship. Ambiguity in the consulting agreement may seem attractive because it offers flexibility in expectations and in addressing needs as they are identified during the consultation process; however, it also poses certain risks. Lack of a clear agreement may feed distrust and provoke suspicion, particularly if the actions of the consultant appear self-serving. Box 5-4 lists suggested components of a consultant agreement.[8] Those new to consulting may want to seek legal advice in developing a template contract for their business.

Codes of Ethics

Lippitt and Lippitt[3] have devised a code of ethics for consultants based on 11 principles:
Responsibility
Competence
Moral and legal standards
Avoidance of misrepresentation
Confidentiality
Client welfare
Announcement of services
Intraprofessional and interprofessional relations
Remuneration
Responsibility toward client organization
Promotional activities

Box 5-4   **COMPONENTS OF A CONSULTING AGREEMENT**

- The nature and scope of the services to be performed
- A statement specifying the consultant's employment status and ownership of any final work product
- The details of payment of compensation and costs
- The duration of the agreement
- In what ways, when, and by whom the agreement can be terminated
- In what ways the work to be performed can be changed and by whom
- Special requirements (covenants) to protect the client, such as the handling of confidential information
- The manner in which any disputes will be handled
- The remedies available (and to whom) for default or failure to perform, as well as remedies that are not available
- The manner in which formal notice is to be given, and how changes in the scope of the assignment are to be recorded

---

Modified from McGonagle J. Vella CM. How to use a consultant in your company. A manager's and executive's guide. New York: John Wiley and Sons; 2001.

APTA Code of Ethics and Guide for Professional Conduct

The ethical principles cited by Lippitt and Lippitt[3] are similar to the expectations of PTs stated in the APTA's *Code of Ethics*.[14] In general, if PT consultants can transfer the ethical standards they are expected to uphold in patient/client management to their consultant/client relationships, they can be relatively confident they are on the right ethical track. The "rules" are the same.

A broader obligation may also exist to provide *pro bono* consulting services. These volunteer experiences also provide the PT with the opportunity to engage in consultation before deciding whether to officially become a consultant.

Even though consulting is one of the oldest roles of the PT, the *Code of Ethics* and the *Guide for Professional Conduct* (GPC) say very little about the consultant role, speaking directly to that role primarily by addressing the PT's responsibility to seek consultation: "A physical therapist shall seek consultation whenever the welfare of the patient will be safeguarded or advanced by consulting those who have special skills, knowledge, and experience" (GPC 11.1).[15] However, many of the principles of patient/client management are also relevant to the work of the consultant. As previously stated, communication, trust, and loyalty are central to the role of the consultant. Clients of PT consultants should expect the consultant to be trustworthy, to maintain confidentiality, and to "make professional judgments that are in the patient's/client's best interests" (GPC 4.1A).[15]

The ethical issues of professional competence, business practices, provision of accurate public information, and consumer protection are especially relevant to the work of the consultant. As suggested by Section 5.1 of the *Guide for Professional Conduct*,[16] PTs who provide consultation should have an appropriate level of experience and expertise for the assigned task: "A physical therapist shall practice within the scope of his/her competence and commensurate with his/her level of education, training, and experience."[15] Although at one time advertising physical therapy services would have been considered unethical, the current version of the *Guide for Professional Conduct* states that PTs may advertise their services as long as this information is accurate (GPC 8.2C, 8.2D).[15]

The ethical dilemma of dual or divided loyalties may manifest differently for consultants than for PTs in patient/client management. For example, a physical therapy consultant may discover that the client is engaging in unethical or illegal activity. Because professionals are accountable to society and are responsible for protecting the public, the consultant must decide whether to report the activity (as required by GPC 9.1C)[16] or protect the client. Recent accounting scandals vividly illustrate the pitfalls for consultants who act solely in the interest of their clients without regard for society as a whole.

Principle 10 of the APTA's *Code of Ethics* seems to suggest that PTs should serve as consultants to the larger society: "Physical therapists shall endeavor to address the health needs of society."[14] The *Guide for Professional Conduct* elaborates upon this as a responsibility to perform *pro bono* public practice (as the practice setting permits) (GPC 10.1) and support efforts to enhance the health of the community (GPC 10.2).[16] Although PTs have an obligation to engage in pro bono and community service activities, physical therapy consultants must remember that these activities may also carry legal liability. PTs frequently rely on malpractice insurance provided by the organization in which they work, and this insurance coverage may not extend to pro bono efforts initiated outside of work.[16]

The types of ethical issues that arise depend on whether the physical therapy consultation occurs as a dimension of patient/client management with an individual or as a contractual arrangement between an external consultant and an organization. Arriaga[17] points out that PTs' everyday efforts to help each other in physical therapy practice are a type of consultation that has the potential to result in serious legal and ethical consequences (see Consulting Scenario 6).

Much of the ethics literature has dealt with the PT's patient/client management role, but relatively little has been written about the PT as consultant. An analysis of peer-reviewed ethics literature from 1970 to 2000 found no such articles that focused on the ethical issues encountered by PTs in the consultant role (see Figure 4-5).[18] This dearth of information indicates a need for further reflection and discussion of the ethical dimensions of this role.

FURTHER THOUGHTS

As a professional with specialized, expert knowledge, any PT has the potential to become a consultant. In fact, consultation may be second nature to PTs because of the consultative nature of the patient/client management role, with which they are so familiar. PTs may choose to supplement their primary physical therapy work by moonlighting as consultants, or they may use their physical therapy knowledge and experience to develop a full-time consulting business. The legal and ethical dimensions of consulting are as complex and challenging as they are in the other roles of the PT.

CONSULTING SCENARIOS

In terms of their professional development and career goals, PTs must determine whether they are comfortable with the entrepreneurial aspects of consulting and the responsibilities inherent in engaging in a different kind of trusting, helping relationship with clients to meet their needs. Many opportunities exist for those with the interest and skills to engage in consultation. The following six scenarios present various aspects of consultation at different levels. They also illustrate typical consulting opportunities, which may help the reader decide whether to pursue the consulting role of the PT.

Consulting Scenario 1

Jill Jankowski has been successful in her independent physical therapy practice, specializing in children with spina bifida. Susie Shaw has asked Jill to act as her consultant as she develops her new pediatric physical therapy practice. Susie tells Jill that she considers her an expert in pediatrics and admires her for her excellent reputation in the community. Jill, who has never served as a consultant before, is flattered to be asked. She tells Susie that she will consider the matter and call her within a week.

- *What should Jill ask herself before she calls Susie with her decision?*

Consulting Scenario 2

An RFP has been announced by Health Care Systems of the Future, Inc., a new health care organization. The goals of phase I of the project are to integrate the physical therapy services of recently merged hospitals and freestanding physical therapy practices and to determine the most effective management strategies for the new system. The plan would be implemented in phase II.

- *Would you submit an RFP? Why or why not?*
- *If you decided to submit the RFP, what components of the project would be most interesting to you?*
- *What aspects of preparing the RFP would be most challenging?*

Consulting Scenario 3

You have volunteered to serve as a consultant to the Metro Area Coalition for Health Care Access for All. You are assigned to develop a proposal that identifies and establishes programs for the uninsured who need physical therapy services, and you are to present your report at the coalition's next board meeting. However, you had expected your role as a consultant to be one of reacting, from a physical therapy standpoint, to ideas and plans presented by someone else.

- *What do you do about this assignment?*

Consulting Scenario 4

ABC electronics has developed an innovative device for analyzing movement disorders. Because you are an expert in movement disorders, the company wants to hire you as a consultant to help design research studies to test the device's reliability and validity; it also wants you to help develop a marketing plan and devise a strategy for getting the device on the market. ABC would like you to be involved in all phases of the process, and your fee would be 10% of the profits earned from the device in the first 3 years.

- *Do you accept the offer? Why or why not?*

Consulting Scenario 5

Village-by-the-Sea Hospital is seeking a PT to develop and implement a new program for improving the physical activity level of cancer survivors. The hospital wants the PT to develop the program's policies, procedures, and protocols, as well as an outcomes evaluation plan; the PT also would be in charge of the program for 6 months while training current staff members. The hospital offers you the position at a fee of $10,000 a month for 6 months. You decide to quit your current job and take advantage of this opportunity.

- *What skills do you need to succeed in this project?*
- *Are you an employee or a consultant?*

Consulting Scenario 6

A PT has been providing physical therapy for a 40-year-old woman with cervical pain for 2 weeks, but the pain has not abated. With the patient's permission, the PT asks another therapist in the same clinic to consult on the case. When the consulting PT begins an examination, the patient complains of jaw pain and leaves without further intervention. At this point, the consulting PT reads the patient's chart and discovers that she has a history of temporomandibular joint problems. After several temporomandibular joint surgeries, the patient sues both PTs for malpractice and negligence.

- *How could this situation have been avoided?*

REFERENCES

1. American Physical Therapy Association. *Interactive guide to physical therapist practice with catalog of tests and measures* (version 1.0). Alexandria, Va: The Association; 2002.
2. Bly RW. *The six-figure consultant: How to start (or jump-start) your consulting career and earn $100,000+ a year.* Chicago: Dearborn; 1998.
3. Lippitt G, Lippitt R. *The consulting process in action* (ed 2). San Francisco: Jossey Bass; 1986.
4. Block P. *Flawless consulting: A guide to getting your expertise used.* San Francisco: Jossey-Bass; 2000.
5. Salacuse JW. *The wise advisor: What every professional should know about consulting and counseling.* Westport, Conn: Praeger; 2000.
6. Maister DH, Green CH, Galford RM. *The trusted advisor.* New York: Free Press; 2000.
7. Fuller GW. *Getting the most out of your consultant: A guide to selection through implementation.* Boca Raton, Fla: CRC Press; 2000.
8. McGonagle J, Vella CM. *How to use a consultant in your company: A managers' and executives' guide.* New York: John Wiley & Sons; 2001.
9. Cohen W. *How to make it big as a consultant* (ed 3). New York: Amacom; 2001.
10. Holtz, H. *Concise guide to being a consultant.* New York: John Wiley & Sons; 1999.
11. Biech E. *The business of consulting: The basics and beyond.* San Francisco: Jossey-Bass/Pfeiffer; 1999.
12. Bermont H. *How to become a successful consultant in your own field.* Rocklin, Calif: Prima; 1997.
13. Hoyt DB. *Start and run a successful independent consulting business: Here's how.* Lincolnwood, Ill: NTC Contemporary; 1997.
14. American Physical Therapy Association. *APTA code of ethics.* Retrieved November 9, 2003, at http://www.apta.org/AM/Template.cfm?Section=Ethics_and_Legal_Issues1&TEMPLATE=/CM/ContentDisplay.cfm&CONTENTID=14342
15. American Physical Therapy Association. *APTA guide for professional conduct.* Retrieved November 9, 2003, at http://www.apta.org/AM/Template.cfm?Section=Ethics_and_Legal_Issues1&TEMPLATE=/CM/ContentDisplay.cfm&CONTENTID=14342
16. Kihn N. Professional liability insurance for the employed PT. *PT Magazine* 1999;7:24-26.
17. Arriaga R. Stories from the front. Part III: Consultation. *PT Magazine* 2000;18:75-76.
18. Swisher LL. A retrospective analysis of ethics knowledge in physical therapy: 1970-2000. *Phys Ther* 2002;82:692-706.

6

The Physical Therapist as Critical Inquirer

Critical inquiry is the process of applying the principles of scientific methods to read and interpret professional literature; participate in, plan, and conduct research; evaluate outcomes data; and assess new concepts and technologies.

– The Interactive Guide to Physical Therapist Practice with Catalog of Tests and Measures version 1.0 (2002)[1]

THE HISTORY OF CRITICAL INQUIRY

From the beginning, the profession of physical therapy has recognized the crucial roles of scientific investigation and critical inquiry. The constitution of the American Women's Physical Therapeutic Association, published in 1921, stated that "the purpose of the Association shall be to establish and maintain a professional and scientific standard for those engaged in the profession of Physical Therapeutics."[2] Also in 1921, *P.T. Review*, the first physical therapy journal, began publication. The aims of the journal were to provide a means by which physicians and reconstruction aides could more easily keep up with each others' work and to preserve the standards and advance the science of the profession.[2]

Mary McMillan acknowledged the importance of this aspect of physical therapy in the preface to the third edition of her textbook, *Therapeutic Exercise and Massage*, published in 1932. She noted that "since the second edition of this book was published there has been a great deal of research in various pathological conditions that are treated by physiotherapeutic measures," and explained that several chapters had been revised so that "the student may be brought in touch with this important phase of physiotherapy work."[3]

This early awareness of the importance of science in the profession has never been lost. However, it has only recently come to the forefront. In the 1975 McMillan Lecture, Helen Hislop lamented that the science of physical therapy was just entering its infancy, even though the profession was over 50 years old. She attributed the difficulty in developing the clinical science of physical therapy to the perception that physical therapy practice was incompatible with the generalizations demanded of science because physical therapists (PTs) treat individual persons.[4] Also, in the early years of the profession, physicians were entrusted with the task of conducting studies related to rehabilitation.

In the 1993 McMillan Lecture, Gary Soderberg again addressed the need for development of the science of physical therapy. He urged academic experts and clinicians to collaborate in contributing to the clinical science of physical therapy and called for an emphasis on clinical research, rather than basic scientific research, to advance the profession.[5]

About the same time, Robertson[6] expressed concern that the profession had failed to accumulate a knowledge base that defined the uniqueness of physical therapy and its scientific merit. In a review of articles in the professional journal *Physical Therapy,* she noted a lack of evidence and coherence among the articles in three topic areas—knee, back, and electrical stimulation—as well as heavy reliance on sources outside the field of physical therapy. She concluded that the profession faces a number of issues in developing its unique knowledge base:

- Lack of agreement on what physical therapy is and what PTs do, as well as on the core knowledge PTs should have
- Lack of understanding of why physical therapy is necessary
- Lack of agreement on terms and concepts
- Lack of clinical literature in the discipline
- Lack of development of relevant theory
- Reliance on medicine and behavioral sciences for a physical therapy knowledge base
- Reliance on informal communication (e.g., personal contacts and oral conference presentations) rather than formal, peer-reviewed information in the practice of physical therapy

In 2003, using the Hedges Project Criteria, Miller, McKibbon, and Haynes[7] conducted a quantitative analysis of articles published in *Physical Therapy,* the *Australian Journal of Physiotherapy, Physiotherapy,* and *Physiotherapy Canada* in 2000 and 2001. On the basis of the criteria that assist in the classification of published research and quality ranking, they concluded that 56% of the 179 articles reviewed were original research and the rest were general discussion or miscellaneous articles. Although the volume of original research appears strong, only 11% of the articles met the Hedges criteria for high-quality evidence suitable for direct application to patient care. This low percentage may be the result of the way quality is defined by the Hedges project, which supports an evidence-based approach to the literature; however, none of the articles addressed etiology, prognosis, or diagnosis or dealt with economics. Miller and colleagues[7] concluded that their findings, although not reflective of all research done by PTs, raised a question: How valuable is some of the research reported in journals to the actual clinical practice of the more than 125,000 PTs who receive at least one professional publication?[7]

More recently, pressures outside the profession have advanced the need to establish the scientific basis of physical therapy clinical practice. Economic decisions based on well-founded scientific information are the trend in health care policy. For example, the demand for outcomes data has been driven by institutional accreditation demands for quality care, which has also increased the demand for scientific support for the health care people receive. As the demand for health care continues to overwhelm available resources, decisions about what to pay for are driven, appropriately or not, by evidence indicating the most effective course for the money spent (see following section and Chapter 4).

Just as with other health care professionals, PTs cannot expect patients and third-party payers to accept on blind faith that PTs do good things and people get better.

Yet, even as the science is emphasized, the impact of the patient-therapist interaction in helping patients achieve their therapeutic goals cannot be underestimated. Because physical therapy remains a "high touch" profession, care must be taken to include research on the human interaction inherent in its practice. As Wolf[8] asks, "Do our patients improve because of the physical interventions we provide, thus affecting their state of well-being, or do our caring and interaction favorably affect patient behaviors, which subsequently motivates them to improve physically?"

Over the past 30 years, the American Physical Therapy Association (APTA) has taken major steps to advance the science of the profession, including formation of the Foundation for Physical Therapy, publication of a clinical research agenda, creation of a clinical research network, and the Hooked on Evidence grass-roots initiative to develop a database for evidence in physical therapy (Boxes 6-1 through 6-4). These efforts contribute to the formation of the physical therapy knowledge base through funding of research, clarification of the primary research questions to be addressed, collaboration among researchers, and collection of evidence to support physical therapy interventions. The need for evidence in physical therapy is an extension of the evidence-based movement in medicine.

EVIDENCE-BASED MEDICINE

According to Sackett et al.,[9] evidence-based medicine (EBM) (or evidence-based practice [EBP] as it applies to other health care professionals) is the integration of the best research evidence with clinical expertise and patient values. Sackett and colleagues define *best research evidence* as clinically relevant research from the basic sciences and patient-centered clinical research that leads to accurate and precise diagnosis and prognostic markers, as well as therapeutic, rehabilitative, and preventive regimens that replace traditional methods with more powerful, accurate, efficacious, and safe practice.[9]

Clinical expertise is the ability to use clinical skills and past experiences to identify each patient's unique health state and diagnosis, as well as the risks and benefits of potential interventions in the context of the patient's personal values and expectations. These values are defined as the unique preferences, concerns,

---

Box **6-1**   THE FOUNDATION FOR PHYSICAL THERAPY

The Foundation for Physical Therapy was established in 1979 as a national, independent, nonprofit corporation to support the research needs of the physical therapy profession in three areas:
- *Scientific research,* to create a solid platform for future clinical research
- *Clinical research,* to assess the efficacy of physical therapy interventions and to help define best practice
- *Health services research,* to assess the effectiveness of physical therapy practice in the emerging health care delivery models

The following are some of the foundation's activities, designed to advance these objectives:
- Assisting clinicians, researchers, and academicians in doctoral programs
- Expanding funding for new researchers
- Supporting clinically relevant research
- Strengthening the Foundation's capacity through fund raising to promote the profession's research agenda

From American Physical Therapy Association. *Foundation for physical therapy.* Retrieved November 9, 2003, at http://www.apta.org/AM/Template.cfm?Section=About_the_Foundation&Template=/TaggedPage/TaggedPage Display.cfm&TPLID=78&ContentID= IDnumber

Box 6-2   **APTA Clinical Research Agenda**

The American Physical Therapy Association (APTA) has established the following research agenda:
1. What is the usefulness of information derived from examination (history/review of systems, tests, and measures) for patient classification that can be used to direct/guide intervention?
    1.1. What measures could be used to classify patients?
    1.2. What are the psychometric properties of tests and measures used for patient classification?
    1.3. What are the psychometric properties of classification systems?
    1.4. How can data best be used for clinical decision making?
    1.5. Are there combinations of measures of impairment and critical levels of function that would predict disability, and, if so, how can we determine them?
2. What is the usefulness of information derived from examination (history, review of systems, tests, and measures) for prognosis?
    2.1. What measures are currently used for prognosis?
    2.2. What are the natural histories of conditions for which physical therapists provide services?
    2.3. What are the relationships among pathology, impairment, functional limitation, and disability?
    2.4. What are the effects of demographic factors (e.g., age, language, race, ethnicity, sex, social history, comorbidity, culture, family/caregiver resources) on the outcome of physical therapy interventions?
3. What are the optimal characteristics of an intervention to achieve a desired effect or outcome (function, satisfaction, cost) for given diagnoses?
    3.1. What is the effectiveness of physical therapy intervention?
    3.2. What is the optimal frequency, intensity, and duration of an intervention to achieve a desired effect or outcome for a given diagnosis?
    3.3. Are there optimal time periods for interventions that influence pathology, impairment, functional limitation, and disability?
    3.4. What is the relative effectiveness of two or more interventions for a particular patient diagnostic classification?
    3.5. What is the optimal combination of interventions to achieve desired patient outcomes?
    3.6. Are there factors that interact with physical therapy interventions, and how do they interact to affect patient outcomes and clinical decision making?
    3.7. What factors predict supply, demand, and need for physical therapy services?

From Clinical Research Agenda Conference Participants. Clinical research agenda for physical therapy. *Phys Ther* 2000;80:499-513.

and expectations of each patient that must be integrated into the professional's decision making.[9]

The popularity of EBP has emerged from clinicians' realization of the following:
*   They need new information on a daily basis.
*   They lack the time to find and assimilate new information.
*   Traditional information resources often are out of date, wrong, and overwhelming in volume.
*   A disparity exists between clinical judgment, which increases with experience, and "current, relevant" information, which decreases with experience.

These problems have diminished with improvements in the means to assess the validity of data, the creation of systematical reviews of health care, the development of evidence-based journals, the creation of electronic systems for electronic retrieval of information, and strategies for lifelong learning.[9] Box 6-5 presents the steps in the EBM process identified by Sackett and co-workers that apply to any professional wanting to engage in EBP.

Box 6-3   **CLINICAL RESEARCH NETWORKS**

A clinical research network (CRN) brings universities, hospitals, clinics, and other institutions together to share resources and work to answer questions important to the physical therapy profession. It provides physical therapists with the opportunity to use a network of resources to conduct research.

The American Physical Therapy Association's Foundation for Physical Therapy put out the first call for letters of intent to develop a clinical research network in June, 2001. The process for funding a CRN had two steps. The Foundation first awarded five applicants planning grants of $5,000 each to develop proposals for CRNs; one of the proposals then was chosen for funding of a single CRN. The selected CRN was funded for a project period of up to 3 years, with a budget for direct costs of up to $500,000 a year.

The first CRN award was made to Carolee J. Winstein, PT, PhD, associate professor in the Department of Biokinesiology and Physical Therapy at the University of Southern California, to establish PTClinResNet, a multisite clinical research network. The goals of Winstein's CRN are to evaluate the effects of muscle-strengthening exercises for the physically disabled, create a lasting structure that will sustain clinical research in physical therapy, and provide education and training opportunities for current and future clinician-researchers in physical therapy.

The site links five premier centers of physical therapy research and practice, which have begun to collaborate on four clinical research projects to assess the effects of strength exercises designed to improve muscle performance and movement skill in patients with the following physical disabilities: adult stroke, pediatric cerebral palsy, shoulder pain in adult paraplegics with spinal cord injury, and orthopedic/low back pain. Having adopted the disablement model as a framework for analysis, PTClinResNet's clinician-researchers will evaluate outcomes resulting from treatment-caused changes in an individual's impairments, functional limitations, and disabilities. Because a common set of valid outcome measures will be used across projects, PTClinResNet's investigators also will be able to compare the effectiveness of treatment across disabilities.

From American Physical Therapy Association. *Clinical research networks.* Retrieved November 9, 2003, at http://www.apta.org/Foundation/News/fpt_newsarchives/CRNInfo. This material is copyrighted, and any further reproduction or distribution is prohibited.

Box 6-4   **HOOKED ON EVIDENCE**

Hooked on Evidence is a national initiative by the American Physical Therapy Association (APTA) to develop a database on the effectiveness of physical therapy interventions. The goal is to give clinicians quick, easy access to the knowledge available from current research.

Hooked on Evidence is a work in progress; it depends on volunteer physical therapists to search the literature on a particular topic, retrieve relevant articles from peer-reviewed literature, summarize the data and findings, and send the review to the APTA for inclusion in the database.

From Coyne C. Getting hooked on Hooked on Evidence. *PT Magazine* 2002;June:34-39.

Box 6-5   **STEPS IN APPLYING EVIDENCE-BASED MEDICINE**

1. Convert the need for information into an answerable question.
2. Track down the best evidence to answer that question.
3. Critically appraise the evidence for validity, impact, and usefulness in clinical practice.
4. Integrate the critical appraisal with clinical expertise and the patient's unique circumstances and values.
5. Evaluate the effectiveness and efficiency of the evidence-gathering process and seek ways to improve these factors.

Questions and concerns raised about evidence-based practice include whether health care professionals actually practice using evidence and whether the outcomes of patient care delivered by EBP professionals differ from those achieved by non-EBP professionals. Being able to access the evidence in clinics and having the skills to assess the evidence critically may be overwhelming for some professionals. Basing broad health care policies on the evidence may conflict with economic policies aimed at reducing the costs of health care. The risk also exists that EBP will prompt an overformalization of clinical guidelines, which will be widely instituted as a substitute for individual clinical judgment.[9] Finally, the high value placed on randomized clinical trials, the gold standard for evidence in medicine, may result in an inappropriate disregard for important, useful information gained through other types of research.

The EBM movement has resulted in the development of several databases for the dissemination of evidence (Box 6-6). These sources of secondary information have resulted in a modification of EBP that Geyman, Deyo, and Ramsey[10] have described as *information mastery* (Figure 6-1). The information mastery approach to answering a question appears to be more efficient because it relies on information already screened for validity and general relevance.

OUTCOMES RESEARCH

Outcomes research is a term applied to different types of health care research.[9] One kind of outcomes research is conducted by analyzing large administrative databases (e.g., Medicare) to explore such issues as utilization, costs, morbidity, and mortality related to certain conditions or interventions. The results of these studies often are used as a complement to evidence-based information. For instance, data on all Medicare patients admitted to hospitals for surgery as a result of osteoarthritis of the hip could be analyzed for differences in length of stay, common secondary conditions that affect discharge disposition, and mortality.

The term *outcomes research* also is used for studies that focus on the end result of health care in terms of health status, disability, and survival. *Effectiveness* studies address how well routine clinical practices work in everyday practice, whereas *efficacy* studies, which are typically conducted as randomized clinical trials in specialty centers with discrete sampling of subjects, address whether clinical practices can

---

Box **6-6   DATABASE SOURCES OF EVIDENCE FOR PRACTICE**

- Cochrane Collaboration (international nonprofit organization providing up-to-date information on health care effects): http://hiru.mcmaster.ca/COCHRANE
- Bandolier (independent U.K. journal by Oxord scientists about evidence-based health care): www.jr2.ox.ac.uk:80/Bandolier
- National Guideline Clearinghouse (database of evidence-based clinical practice guidelines and related documents updated weekly by the Agency for Healthcare Research and Quality in partnership with the American Medical Association and the American Association of Health Plans Foundation): www.ngc.gov
- PEDro (international Physiotherapy Evidence Database providing rapid access to bibliographic details and abstracts of randomized controlled trials, systematic reviews, and evidence-based clinical practice guidelines in physiotherapy): www.pedro.fhs.usyd.edu.au/
- Hooked on Evidence (American Physical Therapy Association's database containing current research evidence on the effeciveness of physical therapy interventions: www.apta.org/hookedonevidence/index.cfm

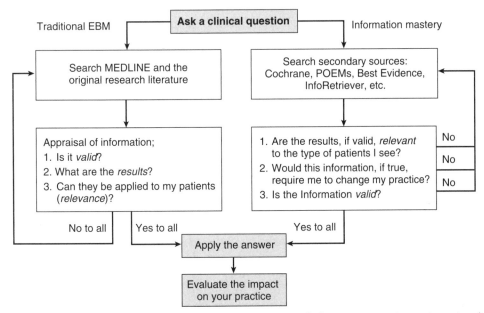

Figure 6-1. Comparison of traditional evidence-based practice (EBP) and information mastery (e.g., patient-oriented evidence that matters [POEM]). (*Modified from Geyman JP, Deyo RA, Ramsey SD. Concepts and approaches. Woburn, Mass: Butterworth-Heinemann; 2000. p.159, Fig 17-2.*)

work in ideal situations. Box 6-7 presents a comparison of effectiveness and efficacy studies of individuals with arthritis.

Broad population-based outcome studies may be conducted by using surveys to gather information from patients on general health and quality of life. Questionnaires that address specific diseases, such as the Arthritis Impact Measurement Scale (AIMS), can also be used.[11] An excellent resource for identifying the wide range of generic and disease-specific instruments is the Quality of Life Instruments Database (QOLID), a web-based database of outcome instruments.[12]

Box 6-7   COMPARISON OF EFFECTIVENESS AND EFFICACY STUDIES OF INDIVIDUALS WITH ARTHRITIS

Question: Is an arthritis education program effective?

Effectiveness Study

A study is designed to determine whether a difference will be seen in the scores on the Arthritis Impact Measurement Scale (AIMS) for 150 participants before and after the subjects complete a 6-week, standardized arthritis education program at three different times of the year in two institutions.

Efficacy Study

A clinical trial is conducted in which 150 randomly selected individuals with bilateral osteoarthritis of the knees are assigned either to a control group or to an experimental group. Both groups are pretested with the AIMS. The experimental group undergoes a 6-week, standardized arthritis education program conducted by a single instructor. At the end of the program, the AIMS scores for both groups are remeasured and compared. The hypothesis is that the AIMS scores of the experimental group will have improved more than those of the control group.

Whose Responsibility is Research?

The subject of who shoulders responsibility for the creation and dissemination of physical therapy knowledge remains a matter of controversy. Certainly physical therapy faculties assume a great deal of responsibility for new knowledge through the academic triad—teaching, scholarship, and service. Doctoral students also meet this need through the traditional dissertation requirement (see Chapter 8). However, the situation of academic researchers functioning independently in academic centers raises concerns about the construction of a profession-wide knowledge base. These individual research agendas are more often driven by personal interest and available funding than by the needs of the profession. As yet, no widespread efforts have been made to engage faculty members to collaborate with clinicians in formulating clinical research projects that could answer both efficacy and effectiveness questions. The Foundation for Physical Therapy's work to create clinical research networks is the first concerted effort to address this issue (see Box 6-3).

The critical inquiry expectations for entry-level PTs pose another educational issue. The criteria for critical inquiry established by the Commission on Accreditation in Physical Therapy Education (CAPTE) are presented in Box 6-8. Several factors influence the way programs actually meet these criteria. The faculty resources available, particularly the time required to supervise formal research studies by individual students, are an important consideration. Some programs emphasize the need to experience the investigative process through a formal thesis process, and require students to conduct formal research studies. The belief is that this requirement teaches students to value research and stimulates interest in advanced studies. Graduate schools also establish expectations. For instance, some colleges require every graduate student to produce a thesis or dissertation to graduate. Despite such emphasis, attitudes about research appear to change after graduation, particularly the individual PT's desire to be involved in research and the priority placed on research in clinical practice.[13]

At a minimum, most physical therapy students are required to demonstrate the ability to use research and to critique new information. The experiences of physical therapy students in critical inquiry, as well as their skill and interest in it, may vary widely. This variation in educational experience may be one factor in the varying quality and quantity of clinical research conducted by physical therapists with patients as subjects.

Box 6-8   Criteria for Critical Inquiry

Critical Inquiry and Clinical Decision Making

3.8.3.8.   Participate in the design and implementation of decision-making guidelines.

3.8.3.9.   Demonstrate clinical decision-making skills, including clinical reasoning, clinical judgment, and reflective practice.

3.8.3.10.   Evaluate published studies related to physical therapy practice, research, and education.

3.8.3.11.   Secure and critically evaluate information related to new and established techniques and technology, legislation, policy, and environments related to patient or client care.

3.8.3.12.   Participate in scholarly activities to contribute to the body of physical therapy knowledge (e.g., case reports, collaborative research).

From the Commission on Accreditation of Physical Therapy Education. *Evaluation criteria for accreditation of education programs for the preparation of physical therapists.* Retrieved November 9, 2003, at http://www.apta.org/Documents/Public/Accred/AppendixB-PT-Criteria.pdf

ROLES OF THE STAFF PHYSICAL THERAPIST IN CRITICAL INQUIRY

The critical inquiry role of the PT may not be as valued or as evident as other roles. For example, in the work of the PT, administrative and education responsibilities become routine, but evidence-based practice and participation in clinical research do not. In 1996, 93.4% of PTs surveyed reported no work-related research activity,[14] and in 2001 PTs reported spending an average of 1% of their time each week on research or critical inquiry.[15]

Critical inquiry and administrative activities may overlap to some degree. For example, of the activities listed in Box 6-8, the development of clinical guidelines (and perhaps critical pathways unique to particular institutions) and the evaluation of outcomes data may be considered administrative functions. Because clinical decision making is a foundation of patient/client management, which in turn closely resembles the consultation process, it also has an administrative aspect.

The following sections explore five remaining aspects of critical inquiry that do not overlap with the PTs' other roles: the PT as (1) a user of research, (2) a publisher of case reports, (3) a collaborator in clinical research studies, (4) an assessor of new concepts and technology, and (5) a research subject.

Application and Critique of Research

PTs can use research in two ways. One approach, evidence-based practice, has been discussed previously. Increasingly, PTs' education gives them the skills to practice evidence-based physical therapy. However, only a small percentage of the practice of physical therapy is supported by evidence; therefore the traditional method, independent critiquing of the literature, continues to be the primary means of updating the specific information needed for clinical practice.

Critique of the literature also is done in journal clubs, which are small groups of practitioners who meet regularly to explore research on a selected topic.[9] These clubs follow one of two models. In one model, which is more conducive to an EBP approach to review of the literature, participants first reach consensus on clinical questions the group has identified. A member is assigned to search the evidence and supply the group with abstracts of reviews or articles that answer the question. The rest of the club members critically appraise the evidence provided, using skills needed in the EBM or information master model (Figure 6-1).

In the more traditional journal club model, participants take turns summarizing assigned journal articles and leading group discussions to critique the studies. Box 6-9 provides guidelines for critiquing a single research report, and Figure 6-2 shows Garrard's matrix method of comparing several research studies on the same topic.[16] These guidelines require some modification for review of qualitative research, and the column titles in the matrix can be modified to address particular types of research. The guidelines and matrix can be used for individual critiques of the literature and as guidelines for journal club discussions. The skills for traditional and evidence-based strategies for critiquing the literature typically are developed in physical therapy school.

Publication of Case Reports

McEwen and colleagues[17] have devised a clinician's guide to writing case reports. They identified the following steps:

Box 6-9   GUIDELINES FOR CRITIQUING RESEARCH REPORTS

To *critique* means to criticize, which means to make judgments, to analyze qualities, and to evaluate the comparative worth of something. A critique must go beyond reporting what the researcher did; it must discuss the *value* of a study to the researcher and to the profession. That is, the researcher must explain why the study does or does not have value. The following questions can serve as a guide to physical therapists in critiquing research reports. Not all questions apply to all studies, and some studies may evoke additional questions.

- What is the purpose of the study?
- What is the question being investigated?
- What type of study is it?
- Who were the subjects? Can the results be applied to the general population of patients?
- What are the merits or limitations of the measurement tools?
- Have all variables been considered? How were extraneous variables controlled?
- What factors could affect the study's reliability and validity? How were they controlled?
- Can the study be duplicated?
- Based on the results, was the question answered?
- Were the statistical tests performed appropriate for the type of data analyzed?
- How do the findings relate to those of other studies?
- Did the researchers discuss the results? What were their conclusions?
- Are methodology limitations addressed?
- Are some conclusions not supported by the study?
- Have suggestions been made for further study? What are yours?
- What is the relevance of the study?
- How will the study affect your practice of physical therapy?
- What is the relevance of the study to the profession?
- How do the results contribute to or test a theory?
- Can you follow the sequence of events in the study?
- Was anything overlooked?
- What would you do next?
- What would you have done differently?
- Is the study report well written?

1. Think. What is the focus of your case?
2. Search the literature. What new insights would your case offer to the knowledge base?
3. Write. Of the following, begin by writing the section you know best but include them all:
   a. Describe the rationale behind the case (introduction)
   b. Describe the patient or situation, the hypothesis, and the intervention (case description)
   c. Describe the outcome (outcomes)
   d. Reflect on what happened (discussion)
4. Submit the case report for publication in a peer-reviewed publication.

These authors view case reports as an extension of routine patient care documentation.[17] The writing process provides clinicians the opportunity to examine clinical observations and reasoning, share their work with a larger audience, and ultimately contribute to improved patient care and the physical therapy knowledge base.

Instructions: Select research reports relevant to the question you seek to answer. Complete a row for each study. Analyze data.*

Author, Title, Journal	Year	Purpose	Variable		Subjects			Data		Comments
			Dependent	Independent	Number	Characteristics	Sample design	Source of instrument	Year(s) collected	

*Column titles will vary depending on type of research designs and data common to studies compared.

Figure 6-2. Model of the matrix method of reviewing research studies. (*From Garrard J.* Health sciences literature review made easy: The matrix method. *Gaithersburg, Md: Aspen; 1999.*)

Collaboration in Clinical Research

According to Fitzgerald and Delitto,[18] research must be done on patients in clinical settings if the physical therapy profession is to document the effectiveness of interventions accurately, validate patient classification systems, and identify prognostic indicators of functional limitations and disability. These researchers identified the following factors as crucial for clinicians conducting clinical research, whether independently, in collaboration with a CRN, or with faculty members in a local physical therapy program[18]:

- Facility or institutional resources
- Patient management issues
- Availability of target patient populations
- Acquisition and maintenance of support from therapists, physicians, and institutional review boards (IRBs)
- Research-related injuries or illness
- Ethical considerations involved in determining whether a protocol must be modified or a project terminated

For PTs, how much clinical research can be done as part of the job and how much must be done in off-work hours depends on whether such research is a goal of the health care organization and whether it is considered a job responsibility of the PT. This is a major challenge facing PTs who seek clinical research opportunities, which may range from simply notifying a collaborating university when a patient is available who meets the criteria for a study subject, to total responsibility for data collection and research design with very little, if any, assistance from academic faculty members.

The logistics of coordinating the IRBs of the collaborating health care and academic institutions can also be time-consuming, and ensuring the privacy and rights of subjects is complicated. Managers of physical therapy services must also be involved in the research planning process to ensure minimal disruption of services to patients who are not part of the study.

Funding of clinical research may need to be supported by internal or external grants. Although many resources (particularly equipment for tests, measures, and interventions) may already be available, the purchase of supplies and equipment solely for clinical research is not likely to be funded through the organization's normal budget. This is particularly true if the results of the research are perceived to be more important to the profession than to the organization. The preparation of proposals requesting funding is another potential barrier to clinicians interested in conducting research that demands financial support. Case reports, which require little more than the time needed to write down what has already occurred with a patient, have the added advantage of being inexpensive to produce.

Robertson[19] reports that fewer than 1% of clinicians publish investigative work. As the author notes, the barriers to clinical research must be overcome if PTs are to transform the implicit, individual knowledge inherent in their expertise into explicit knowledge that contributes to the broader body of knowledge in physical therapy.[19]

Assessment of New Concepts and Technology

Hislop[4] cautioned PTs against conferring honor and respect on clinical methodologies or theories that lack a scientific basis. This is particularly good advice for PTs choosing continuing education courses or selecting among the many types of equipment for tests, measures, and interventions that technological advances have created. At the least, PTs must use common sense to distinguish between marketing promotions and scientific information that supports the class or equipment. "Buyer beware" applies to professional as well as personal buying. Box 6-10 presents guidelines for assessing classes and products.

Harris[20] recommended a strategy for determining the scientific merit of nontraditional physical therapy treatments that can also be applied to a wide range of interventions, tests, and measures. The PT should determine whether

1. The theories underlying the intervention or instrument are supported by valid anatomical and physiological evidence
2. The intervention or instrument is designed for a specific type of patient population
3. Potential side effects are presented
4. Studies from peer-reviewed journals that support the intervention's or instrument's efficacy are provided
5. The supportive peer-reviewed studies include well-designed, randomized, controlled clinical trials or well-designed single-subject experimental studies
6. The proponents of the intervention or instrument are open and willing in discussing its limitations

Box **6-10**   QUESTIONS TO HELP ASSESS PRODUCTS AND COURSES

Products

- Does the equipment produce the physiological effects intended or promised? How do you know?
- Will the equipment improve the intended treatment outcome?
- How does the equipment accommodate the caseload?
- What is the manufacturer's reputation?
- Is the equipment user friendly? What are the training requirements and costs?
- How does the price compare to that of similar equipment? What are the service and warranty costs?
- Can references be obtained from satisfied customers, and can others who have used the equipment be contacted?

Courses

- Does the content presented have a scientific basis? Are the theories underlying the content identified?
- Does the course have a clearly defined purpose or rationale? Are learning outcomes stated, and are the objectives reasonable for the duration and description of the program?
- Are the learning outcomes compatible with professional development or the improvement goals of course participants?
- Are the faculty members qualified to teach the course?
- Are the target audience and level of instruction clearly defined? Is the number of participants appropriate for achievement of course goals?
- How does the course compare with other programs that have a similar content in terms of cost, goals, and the credentials of speakers?
- Can previous students be contacted for endorsement of the course?

Modified from American Physical Therapy Association. Be a smart consumer. *PT Magazine* August 1993:10-22; and American Physical Therapy Association. *APTA guidelines for evaluating continuing education programs.* Retrieved November 9, 2003, at http://www.apta.org/Education/Continuing_Education/Guidelines_CEProgs

Serving as a Research Subject

PTs may be called upon to serve as subjects in research studies. In addition to a commitment to thoughtful, honest data collection, the decision to participate involves consideration of the following:

- Value of the study to physical therapy
- Integrity of the research design
- Time required to participate
- Length of time to complete the study
- Ability to sustain interest and objectivity to project completion

Other types of research, such as survey research; Delphi studies, which are a type of consensus process; and other qualitative designs may be less time-consuming although they require the same review to determine their value and importance and the same commitment to honesty in responses.

ETHICAL AND LEGAL ISSUES IN CRITICAL INQUIRY

In the critical inquiry role, PTs must fulfill their responsibility to society to protect research subjects and their responsibility to individuals to protect their rights. In this section these concepts are viewed from several perspectives, including the APTA's *Code of Ethics* and *Guide for Professional Conduct,* the protection of human subjects in research, the requirements of IRBs, the differences between patients and research subjects, the responsibilities of clinical researchers, and the ethical challenges of EBP.

APTA Code of Ethics and Guide for Professional Conduct

The APTA's *Guide for Professional Conduct* addresses research through the *Code of Ethics.*[21,22] Principle 5 of the code places a duty on the PT to "maintain and promote high standards for physical therapy practice, education, and research."[22] Section 6.5A states that a PT "participating in research shall abide by ethical standards governing protection of human subjects and dissemination of results." The next section (6.5B) oldigates PTs to "support research activities that contribute knowledge for improved patient care,"[22] and Section 6.5C directs PTs to report unethical acts "in the conduct or presentation of research."[22] Other sections of the *Guide for Professional Conduct* (GPC) and the *Code of Ethics* (COE) specifically address the issues of truthfulness (GPC 2.2), autonomy and consent (GPC 2.4), and compliance with laws and regulations (COE 3). Using and providing accurate, relevant information (COE 8) are also responsibilities of the researcher.[21,22]

Protection of Human Subjects

The myriad laws and regulations that establish the protection of human research subjects originated in the Nuremberg Code of 1947, a reaction to the participation of physicians in inhumane experimentation on human subjects during the Nazi Holocaust. The Nuremberg Code outlined the basic principles of ethical research on humans: voluntary participation; the disclosure of risks to subjects; a design that merits any risks the subjects face; the avoidance of injury and suffering; the prohibition of studies that put subjects at risk of death or disability; the right of subjects to terminate participation; the balancing of risks against societal benefits; and the responsibilities of the researcher.[23,24] Implicit in the Nuremberg guidelines is a commitment to informed consent that is grounded in the ethical principle of autonomy. Box 6-11 summarizes the basic ethical principles governing research.

Institutional Review Boards

Over the past half century, federal regulations to ensure protection of human subjects have developed continually, culminating in the Common Rule of 1991 (Title 45 of the Code of Federal Regulations, Part 46).[23] The Common Rule requires all institutions that receive federal funding to ensure that the research is ethical and that human subjects are protected. IRBs are the mechanism by which institutions determine whether the benefit to society from a research study warrant the risk to individual subjects in the study.

An important feature of this process is the use of IRBs to review research before it is implemented. In practice, this means that an individual who wants to conduct a

---

Box **6-11**   E╍╍╍╍HICAL P╍╍╍╍INCIPLES OF H╍╍╍╍MAN R╍╍╍╍SEARCH

The Belmont Report: Ethical Principles and Guidelines for the Protection of Human Subjects was published in 1979. It provides the philosophical underpinnings for current laws governing research with human subjects. Unlike the *Nuremberg Code* and the *Helsinki Declaration,* which set forth "guidances" or "rules," the *Belmont Report* establishes three fundamental ethical principles: respect for persons, beneficence, and justice. Although other important principles sometimes apply to research, these three provide a comprehensive framework for ethical decision making in research involving human subjects.

1. The principle of *respect for persons* acknowledges the dignity and autonomy of individuals and directs that those with diminished autonomy be given special protection. This principle requires that subjects give informed consent to participation in research. Because of their potential vulnerability, certain subject populations are provided with additional protections; these include live human fetuses, children, prisoners, the mentally disabled, and people with severe illnesses.
2. The principle of *beneficence* requires researchers to protect individuals by maximizing anticipated benefits and minimizing possible harm. The design of a study and its risks and benefits, therefore, must be examined carefully. In some cases this means that alternative ways must be found to obtain the benefits sought from the research. Risks must always be justified by the expected benefits of the research.
3. The principle of *justice* requires that subjects be treated fairly. For example, subjects should be carefully and equitably chosen to ensure that certain individuals or classes of individuals (e.g., prisoners, the elderly, or the poor) are neither systematically selected nor excluded unless scientifically or ethically valid reasons exist for doing so. Also, unless an exception is carefully justified, research should not involve individuals from groups that are unlikely to benefit from subsequent applications of the results.

Each of these principles carries strong moral force, and difficult ethical dilemmas arise when they conflict. Unfortunately, careful, thoughtful application of the principles does not always achieve a clear resolution. Nevertheless, researchers must understand and apply these principles to help ensure that people who agree to be experimental subjects are treated in a respectful and ethical manner.

From National Institutes of Health. *Guidelines for the conduct of research involving human subjects at the National Institutes of Health: Regulations and guidelines of the National Institutes of Health* (revised 3/2/95). Retrieved November 9, 2003, at http://ohsr.od.nih.gov/guidelines.php3#x_app2

research study must prepare an application that describes the proposed study, outlining the nature of the research and describing the risks and benefits, the ways in which subjects will be recruited and informed consent will be obtained, and other relevant information. Although most researchers lament the volume of paperwork involved, the review process provides another layer of safety to ensure that the rights of subjects have received adequate attention.

Subjects vs. Patients

A patient should reasonably expect that health care providers will attempt to place the individual's interests first, respect confidentiality, be truthful, disclose relevant information, respect individual and cultural differences, and collaborate with the patient in achieving goals. After all, the intent of the PT in the patient/client management role is to promote the best interests of the patient.

The role of the PT in critical inquiry is markedly different, because the primary intent of the researcher is to advance knowledge through work with subjects. (The passivity of the term *subject* has led some researchers, especially qualitative researchers, to recommend use of the term *participant*.) The extensive regulations protecting research subjects point up the inherent differences between patients and subjects.

Responsibilities of Clinical Researchers

The differences between patients and subjects may create a sense of divided loyalty or conflict of interest for clinicians involved in research. When considering whether to participate in a clinical research study, practitioners should ask themselves these questions:

- Do patients who agree to participate in a study truly feel free not to enroll, given the perceived power of the PT over patients?
- Does the dual role of patient/subject create obstacles to keeping the patient's interests paramount?
- Can the PT maintain "typical" therapist-patient interactions or relationships to avoid biasing the results of the study?

Besides protecting human subjects, PTs who participate in clinical research have a responsibility to report results honestly and accurately, to report both positive and negative results, and to comment constructively on research literature. The APTA has developed a policy statement that provides guidance on the issue of integrity in research.[25] The recent EBP movement presents additional challenges.

Ethics and Evidence-Based Practice

Investigation of the effectiveness of physical therapy interventions is undeniably necessary and potentially stands to benefit patients, clients, and society. For this reason, most PTs have embraced the concept of evidence-based practice. However, little attention has been paid to the ethical assumptions and implications of the dominant model of EBP, the version proposed by Sackett et al. For example, the following questions deserve further attention[26]:

- Does the emphasis of EBP on outcomes and results commit physical therapy to a consequentialist (ends-based) ethic? (A consequentialist ethic emphasizes the consequences or ends of actions over duties, obligations, rights, or virtues.)

- How can human rights and dignity be protected if a consequentialist framework is adopted for decision making?
- Should the focus be on evidence or on patients? Does the term *evidence-based practice* shift attention away from patient-centered care?
- Does the focus on evidence rather than the patient represent a return to paternalism, especially since researchers design studies with little or no input from patients and clients?
- Because some outcomes are difficult to measure (e.g., pain, quality of life),[26] does the Sackett model essentially commit PTs to gathering evidence about the "easy" questions?
- Are individuals with chronic disabilities at a disadvantage with a model that allocates resources based on evidence of effectiveness?
- Does EBP value majority concerns over minority concerns, given that obtaining adequate samples for randomly controlled studies of smaller groups is much more difficult?
- Will Sackett's narrow definition of *evidence* advance the interests of patients and clients and the profession of physical therapy? (Using Sackett's definition, a researcher would have difficulty obtaining "best" evidence about questions regarding social science issues, ethics, or values, because the variables of investigation are not amenable to the randomly controlled trial, the gold standard research design.)

This is not to suggest that physical therapy should abandon the goal of providing evidence for the effectiveness of treatments. Rather, the profession should work toward a model for evaluating evidence that (1) includes all questions relevant to physical therapy; (2) places the interests of patients at the center; (3) recognizes the importance of qualitative and social science methods; (4) encourages partnerships between patients and PTs in research as well as in patient/client management, and (5) acknowledges the importance of ethics and values in health care.

Critical Inquiry Role in the Ethics Literature

Although it has not been explored as extensively as the PT's role in patient/client management, the critical inquiry role has been the subject of a handful of peer-reviewed articles; from 1970 to 2000, 9.9% of peer-reviewed publications dealt with critical inquiry (see Figure 4-5).[27] Informed consent and protection of human subjects also were frequent topics.

FURTHER THOUGHTS

Of all the roles of the PT, critical inquiry is perhaps the most underdeveloped yet the most critical for advancement of the profession. It also is the role that requires the most initiative from the PT, because employers may not be convinced of the need for critical inquiry. At the least, PTs have a responsibility to be skilled users of research through traditional or evidence-based methods. Opportunities for publishing case reports, collaborating with academic and clinical researchers, assessing new concepts and technology, participating in clinical research networks (CRNs), and serving as research subjects offer PTs the means to contribute to the profession's body of knowledge. PTs who seek professional opportunities as researchers typically do so through doctoral studies and academic appointments. As with other professions, the PT engaged in clinical research must embrace the ethical responsibilities inherent in such work. Professional issues related to critical inquiry are presented in the following case scenarios.

CASE SCENARIOS

Case Scenario 1

You work for a large, multicenter health care system that includes six physical therapy outpatient satellite centers. Through the information systems used for documentation and billing, you have access to more than 10,000 patients who have received outpatient physical therapy services over the past few years. Assume that you can access this data while maintaining the privacy of these discharged patients.
- *What research question or questions could you pose?*
- *What data would you use to answer that question (or those questions)?*
- *What are the disadvantages or limits of this type of research?*

Case Scenario 2

Your boss has asked you to organize a journal club for the six PTs who work in acute and subacute care units in your hospital.
- *What plan for a journal club would you present at your next staff meeting?*

Case Scenario 3

You have job opportunities at four physical therapy centers in the city where you want to relocate. The hours, salary, benefits, and work environment are essentially equal. However, you also are considering the role research plays at each center. Center One is part of a clinical research network, and you would have the opportunity to take part in data collection for a variety of projects in which you are interested. At Center Two, the staff includes three people who have conducted independent clinical research and who have a strong record of publication of their work. The job expectation is that you eventually would develop your own research agenda and follow their lead. Center Three is known for its commitment to professional development, and it supports staff member advancement through scholarships to the local university for graduate study. Several of the center's staff members have pursued doctoral studies and now have academic positions at the affiliated university. Center Four focuses on the delivery of high-quality care and conducts outcomes studies, but no plans have been made to involve you in those studies.
- *Which position do you accept? Why?*

Case Scenario 4

As a PT, you own an independent practice specializing in the care of people with complex regional pain syndrome. A member of the physical therapy faculty at the university about 90 miles away has asked you to participate in a study to determine the effectiveness of a new technique for treating complex regional pain syndrome. You are very excited about the possibility of participating in a project that may improve the outcomes for people with this condition.
- *What questions do you need to ask the faculty member before agreeing to participate and offering your patients the opportunity to be subjects in the study?*

QUESTIONS FOR REFLECTION

1. Select a research report published in *Physical Therapy* in the past 6 months and critique it. Pose a question that is raised as a result of your critique.
2. Identify three or four other research reports on the same topic and use the matrix method to compare the studies. What is your conclusion?
3. Go to any evidence-based medicine database of your choice and answer the question addressed in the studies you critiqued. How were these approaches to enhancing your clinical practice with new information different? How were they the same? How do you decide which one to use when new questions arise?
4. Find a recent issue of *PT Magazine* and select an advertisement for any physical therapy product and for any continuing education course that are of interest to you. What additional information would you seek before buying the product or enrolling in the course? Prepare a list of questions, and call to obtain this information. Based on the answers you were given, would you buy the product or enroll in the course? Why or why not?
5. Choose an issue of *Physical Therapy* and select a case report to read. How does it differ from research reports? What is your critique of the case report?

REFERENCES

1. American Physical Therapy Association. *Interactive guide to physical therapist practice with catalog of tests and measures* (version 1.0). Alexandria, Va: The Association; 2002.
2. American Physical Therapy Association. *The beginnings: Physical therapy and the APTA*, Alexandria, Va: The Association; 1979.
3. McMillan M. *Therapeutic exercise and massage* (3rd ed). Philadelphia: WB Saunders; 1932.
4. Hislop HJ. Tenth Mary McMillan Lecture: The not-so-impossible dream. *Phys Ther* 1975;55:1069-1080.
5. Soderberg GL. Twenty-seventh Mary McMillan Lecture: On passing from ignorance to knowledge. *Phys Ther* 1993;73:797-808.
6. Robertson VJ. Research and the cumulation of knowledge in physical therapy. *Phys Ther* 1995;75:223-236.
7. Miller PA, McKibbon KA, Haynes RB. A quantitative analysis of research publications in physical therapy journals. *Phys Ther* 2003;83:123-131.
8. Wolf SL. Thirty-third Mary McMillan Lecture: Look forward, walk tall: Exploring our "what if" questions. *Phys Ther* 2002;82:1108-1119.
9. Sackett DL, Haynes BM, Straus SE, et al. *Evidence-based medicine* (2nd ed). New York: Churchill Livingstone; 2000.
10. Geyman JP, Deyo RA, Ramsey SD. *Evidence-based clinical practice: Concepts and approaches.* Woburn, Mass: Butterworth-Heinemann; 2000.
11. MAPI Research Institute. *QOLID (quality of life instruments database): Arthritis Impact Measurement Scale.* Retrieved November 9, 2003, at http://www.qolid.org/
12. MAPI Research Institute. *QOLID (quality of life instruments database).* Retrieved November 9, 2003, at http://www.qolid.org/
13. Connolly BH, Lupinnaci NS, Bush AJ. Changes in attitudes and perceptions about research in physical therapy among professional physical therapist students and new graduates. *Phys Ther* 2001; 81:1127-1134.
14. American Physical Therapy Association. *1996 practice profile report.* Alexandria, Va: The Association; 1996.

15. American Physical Therapy Association. *APTA 2001 practice profile survey: Results.* Retrieved November 9, 2003, at http://www.apta.org/pdfs/research/2001PracticeProfileResults.pdf

16. Garrard J. *Health sciences literature review made easy: The matrix method.* Gaithersburg, Md: Aspen; 1999.

17. McEwen I, editor. *Writing case reports: A how-to manual for clinicians.* Fairfax, Va: American Physical Therapy Association; 1996.

18. Fitzgerald GK, Delitto A. Considerations for planning and conducting clinic-based research in physical therapy. *Phys Ther* 2001;81:1446-1454.

19. Robertson VJ. Epistemology, private knowledge and real problems. *Physiotherapy* 1996;82:534-539.

20. Harris SR. How should treatments be critiqued for scientific merit? *Phys Ther* 1996;76:175-181.

21. American Physical Therapy Association. *APTA guide for professional conduct.* Retrieved October 27, 2004, at http://www.apta.org/AM/Template.cfm?

22. American Physical Therapy Association. *APTA code of ethics.* Retrieved December 8, 2004, at http//:www.apta.org/AM/Template.cfm?

23. National Institutes of Health. *Guidelines for the conduct of research involving human subjects at the National Institutes of Health: Regulations and guidelines of the National Institutes of the Health* (revised 3/2/95). Retrieved November 9, 2003, at http://ohsr.od.nih.gov/guidelines.php3#x_app2

24. Swisher LL, Krueger-Brophy C. *Legal and ethical issues in physical therapy.* Woburn, Mass: Butterworth-Heinemann; 1998.

25. American Physical Therapy Association. *Integrity in research policy* [BOD 11-01-12-06]. Retrieved November 9, 2003, at www.apta.org/governance/governance_5/BODpolicies/board_policies1

26. Kerridge I, Lowe M, Henry D. Ethics and evidence-based medicine. *BMJ* 1998;316:1151-1153.

27. Swisher LL. A retrospective analysis of ethics knowledge in physical therapy: 1970-2000. *Phys Ther* 2002;82:592-706.

7

The Physical Therapist as Educator

Education is the process of imparting information or skills and instructing by precept, example, and experience so that individuals acquire knowledge, master skills, or develop competence. In addition to instructing patients/clients as an element of intervention, physical therapists may engage in education activities such as planning and conducting academic education, clinical education, and continuing education programs; planning and conducting educational programs for local, state, and federal agencies; planning and conducting programs for the public to increase awareness of issues in which physical therapists have expertise.

— The Interactive Guide to Physical Therapist Practice with Catalog of Tests and Measures version 1.0 (2002)[1]

THE HISTORY OF PHYSICAL THERAPY EDUCATION

In 1917 the U.S. Army began to plan for the physical rehabilitation of the legions of injured soldiers returning home from World War I. In 1918 Mary McMillan was granted a leave of absence from the Army to develop one of seven emergency training programs for reconstruction aides, the forerunners of today's physical therapists (PTs), at Reed College in Portland, Oregon. In 1919 McMillan became head of the reconstruction aide training program at Walter Reed General Hospital, and in 1921 she wrote *Massage and Therapeutic Exercise,* the first textbook on physical therapy. Figure 7-1 presents an excerpt from the third edition of the text, published in 1932.[2]

McMillan left the Army in 1920 to take a position in Boston. While there, she and Dr. Frank Granger, a physician with whom she had worked in the reconstruction aide project, developed graduate programs for PTs through the Harvard Graduate Medical School.

Meanwhile, as the need for rehabilitative services in the military dwindled, many of the reconstruction aide projects were discontinued, and a jumble of programs appeared to prepare physiotherapists to meet the needs of the civilian population. Some of these programs were based in universities whereas others were based in hospitals.

212 THERAPEUTIC EXERCISE

Flexibility is attained by increasing the rate of speed of the free exercises. Endurance is developed by taking long periods of exercise at a time without an interval of rest. Co-ordination is emphasized in many of the arm leg and trunk exercises.

Rhythm has an important place. In many instances the older methods of precision are substituted by rhythmical exercises and the military note of command in the Swedish system is entirely lacking in the more recently developed system known as "Danish Gymnastics."

Many of the exercises for increasing Flexibility and co-ordination in the Danish system are helpful in therapeutic work. They have to be chosen with discrimination and tried out most carefully.

The subject of therapeutic exercise is a larger one than has been generally considered. It should not be confined to orthopedics or to any one branch of medicine. The intelligent use of therapeutic exercises is a valuable asset in pre- and postoperative work, in many medical cases, in various types of paralysis, and in cardiovascular conditions. An intelligent understanding of the application of therapeutic exercises used conjointly with massage is of great importance. In cases of low back conditions improved posture may have a direct bearing on the strain imposed on the ligaments of the low back. In subdeltoid bursitis the time to begin voluntary exercises, such as wall creeping....

Figure 7-1. Excerpt from *Massage and Therapeutic Exercise*, the first physical therapy textbook, written by Mary McMillan. *(From McMillan M. Massage and therapeutic exercise, 3rd ed. Philadelphia: WB Saunders; 1932. p. 212.)*

It became clear that the educational requirements for physiotherapists needed to be standardized, and in 1929 the American Physiotherapy Association suggested a curriculum to be used as a minimum standard for schools of physiotherapy (Box 7-1).[3] Given the prolonged struggle of the profession at the end of the century to implement educational requirements beyond the baccalaureate level, it is striking that these 1929 standards suggested a postbaccalaureate curriculum with strong ties to medicine that could be completed in 9 months. In 1930, 11 schools met or exceeded these standards, as determined by the Council on Medical Education and Hospitals of the American Medical Association (AMA)(Box 7-2).[4]

From 1957 to 1976, the American Physical Therapy Association (APTA) collaborated with the AMA to approve physical therapy education programs. In 1977 the APTA'S Commission on Accreditation in Physical Therapy Education (CAPTE) became the recognized accrediting body for physical therapy educational programs. By January, 2003, the list of CAPTE-accredited programs included 204 PT and 459 physical therapist assistant (PTA) programs.[5]

The criteria for accreditation were modified in 1996 to incorporate language and concepts from the APTA's *Guide to Physical Therapist Practice*[1] and the *Normative Model of Physical Therapist Professional Education*.[6] In theory, accreditation is a voluntary process, the purpose of which is quality improvement. In reality, however,

Box 7-1   THE FIRST RECOMMENDED PHYSICAL THERAPY CURRICULUM

The American Physiotherapy Association has a suggested curriculum as a minimum standard for schools of physical therapy.

Length of Course

9 months including 1200 hours, 33 hours per week.

Entrance Requirements

Graduates of recognized schools of physical education, or
Graduates of recognized schools of nursing.

Subjects to Be Taught by Members of the Medical Profession

Anatomy
Physiology
Surgical observation
Orthopedics
Pathology

Major Subjects	Theory	Practice	Total
Anatomy			300
Physiology	36	36	72
Orthopedics	36	36	72
Muscle training	36	72	108
Corrective exercise	36	72	108
Massage	18	72	90
Electrotherapy	18	54	72
Minor Subjects			
Pathology	36		36
Surgical observation		36	36
Principles of apparatus	6		6
Chemistry	27	54	81
Physics	27	54	81
Kinesiology	36		36
Ethics	6		6
Psychology	18		18
Light therapy	18		18
Hydrotherapy	6	18	24
Mechanotherapy		6	6
Thermotherapy	1	2	3

From the American Physical Therapy Association. *The beginnings: Physical therapy and the APTA.* Alexandria, Va: APTA; 1979. pp. 48-49. This material is copyrighted, and any further reproduction or distribution is prohibited.

the link between accreditation and licensure means that participation in the accreditation process becomes mandatory. To be eligible for licensure as a PT or PTA, a person must be a graduate of a CAPTE-accredited physical therapy program.

Because the profession emerged from a variety of settings, a persistent challenge in physical therapy education has been the development of programs at various educational levels. Before the term *allied health* was popularized during the congressional deliberations that led to passage of the *Allied Health Professions Personnel Training Act* of 1967, physical therapy education was based in hospitals or universities. Passage of the Personnel Training Act produced the new concept of unifying the various allied health disciplines into academic units with a single administration.

Box 7-2   FIRST APPROVED SCHOOLS OF PHYSICAL THERAPY

New Haven School of Physiotherapy, New Haven, Connecticut
Philadelphia Orthopedic Hospital, Philadelphia, Pennsylvania
Los Angeles Children's Hospital, Los Angeles, California
Northwestern Medical School, Chicago, Illinois
Battle Creek Sanitarium, Battle Creek, Michigan
Harvard Medical School, Courses 441 and 442, Boston, Massachusetts
Walter Reed General Hospital, Washington, D.C.
Tacoma General Hospital, Tacoma, Washington
Hospital School of the University of Michigan, Lansing, Michigan
Hospital School of the University of Wisconsin, Madison, Wisconsin
Boston School of Physical Education, Boston, Massachusetts
Stanford University Hospital, Palo Alto, California
Hospital for Ruptured and Crippled, New York, New York
College of William and Mary, Williamsburg, Virginia

From Murphy W. *Healing the generations: A history of physical therapy and the American Physical Therapy Association.* Alexandria, Va: APTA; 1995.

The federal funding made available by the law allowed many freestanding physical therapy schools to become part of the new colleges of allied health, which typically awarded the baccalaureate degree.

Classification of physical therapy as an allied health profession remains the trend today. Some have suggested that this is detrimental to the development of the profession, because the allied health disciplines include a diverse group of degree programs. Also, this designation perpetuates the concept of physical therapy as a subsidiary of medicine rather than an autonomous profession. Consequently, the movement away from affiliation with the AMA for program accreditation had been set back, resulting in some loss of autonomy.[4]

However, current accreditation policies reflect the effort to continue the move toward autonomous practice. In January, 2002, CAPTE began accrediting only programs that awarded postbaccalaureate degrees. With many programs making the transition to the postbaccalaureate level, the APTA issued this new vision statement: "By 2020, physical therapy will be provided by physical therapists who are doctors of physical therapy."[7] Meanwhile, the awarding of multiple degrees for entry-level practice continues. This situation arose after World War II, when PTs held degrees at the baccalaureate, master's, and certificate levels; currently, most practicing PTs hold bachelor of science (B.S.) degrees, but new graduates hold the master's or doctor of physical therapy (DPT) degree.

CONTEMPORARY EDUCATIONAL ROLES OF THE PHYSICAL THERAPIST

PTs serve as educators at a variety of levels, from patient instruction to teaching as tenured professors. Co-workers, physical therapy students, and PTA students in both the classroom and clinical practice, as well as other groups of professional and lay people, are potential audiences. Teaching opportunities, therefore, can take a number of forms:

- Informal, short classes
- In-service courses for other staff members to update information or provide training for specific skills

- Continuing education courses
- Clinical instruction (e.g., clinical instructor or center coordinator of clinical education)
- Academic programs (e.g., adjunct faculty member, academic coordinator of clinical education, or full-time tenure track faculty member)

Instruction of Patients

Patient instruction is a primary component of every physical therapy intervention. It is the process of informing, teaching, or training patients (or families and caregivers) in techniques that promote and optimize physical therapy services. This instruction may cover a number of topics, such as the patient's current condition and the related impairments, functional limitations, and disabilities; plans of care; the need for enhanced motor performance; a transition to a different treatment setting; risk factors; or the need for health, wellness, and fitness programs.[1]

Patient instruction may be integrated into a treatment session or provided as a separate, formal intervention (Box 7-3). For example, during an exercise program, PTs may instruct the patient in the principles of exercise, as well as the importance of exercise to overall health, or devote an entire treatment session to training a caregiver in home exercises and transfer techniques or answering questions about a patient's condition.

One-on-one instruction is a patient care skill expected of all PTs, and it lays the foundation for goal setting and instructional strategies in other teaching venues.

Teaching Roles Beyond Patient Care

Many PTs are assigned or volunteer to make presentations as part of their job responsibilities. Such a teaching assignment may be a one-time only session, or it might be a component of a continuing training program. Examples of such presentations include

- In-service classes for physical therapy or other staff members to present new information or update skills (e.g., updating interventions for the hemiplegic shoulder or reviewing current procedural terminology [CPT] coding skills)

Box 7-3 **EXAMPLE PLAN OF CARE WITH INSTRUCTIONAL INTERVENTIONS**

Patient Learning Goals
- Patient will demonstrate the ability to engage in a home exercise program twice a day.
- Patient will discuss the promotion of the healing of tissues after total knee arthroplasty.
- Patient will devise a plan to protect joints in other involved body parts.
- Caregiver will demonstrate the ability to transfer patient with moderate assistance.
- Caregiver will develop a plan to reduce the risk of falls in the home.

Instructional Interventions
- Instruct the patient in the home exercise program and in connective tissue healing and joint protection principles.
- Train the caregiver in transfer techniques.
- Teach the caregiver how to identify obstacles that create safety risks in the home and provide tips for eliminating them.

- Job training programs (e.g., instructing nurses' aides in body mechanics and in assisting patients with ambulation regimens)
- Educational programs for groups of patients with common needs (e.g., making a presentation on skin protection to the local diabetes association support group, or teaching spouses of stroke survivors strategies for increasing their loved one's activity level)
- Public service presentations (e.g., making presentations in public schools or to service-based organizations about the physical therapy profession or movement disorders)

These educational presentations involve the same degree of preparation as other types of instruction[8] (Box 7-4).

Box 7-4   **Tips for Giving a Good Presentation**

The cardinal rule of a good presentation is this—Get up, say what you have to say, and sit down. Steps to take in achieving this goal include

1. Determine the single overriding communications objective, that is, the single purpose of your presentation.
2. Make sure you know why you are making the presentation: to sell, to teach, to motivate, or to persuade.
3. Always plan what you are going to say.
4. Each visual should support the purpose of the presentation; avoid complex data and excessive information. Less information means less distraction. As a general guideline, use five slides in a 10-minute presentation.
5. Use graphics, rather than lots of text, to portray concepts.
6. Hand out more material than you say and say more than you show.
7. Keep handouts simple and consistent; avoid using multiple colors, textures, and fonts. An audience that is too aware of color, typeface, and layout will be less aware of the point of the presentation.
8. Make your point without overwhelming the audience.
9. A simple, clear presentation made in a quiet, confident, and friendly manner results in greater retention of the material.
10. Pay attention to the background colors you use in your presentation materials because they can affect the mood of the audience.
    - Blue signifies a conservative, credible approach to information. It has a calming effect and elicits feelings of trust and safety. White or yellow text on a blue background is the easiest to read.
    - Green stimulates audience interaction and is best for training and educational presentations. It suggests immovable, analytical, precise, opinionated.
    - Red is stimulating. It increases the heart rate and audience enthusiasm and therefore is the color of choice to persuade or motivate to act.
    - Black evokes a sense that the audience has no choice; it should be used for information that cannot be changed (e.g., financial reports).
    - Gray suggests a lack of commitment to the content.
    - Yellow evokes a sense of optimism but is difficult to use with most text colors.
    - Brown leads to audience passivity; it suggests that the content is solid and permanent.
    - Violet implies a magical or mystical quality of the content; it should be used when the material is meant to be entertaining.

Modified from course materials of R. Elliott Churchill, Information management in public health settings, presented at the University of South Florida College of Public Health, Tampa, Fla, Summer 2001.

Teaching Opportunities in Clinical Education

Clinical faculty members, who train and supervise students at clinical education sites, typically work one-on-one with a PT or PTA student. In physical therapy education, the two kinds of clinical faculty members are the clinical instructor (CI) and the center coordinator of clinical education (CCCE).[6] CIs instruct and supervise students directly during clinical education. They are responsible for providing a sound clinical education and for assessing students' performance based on entry-level practice expectations.

After at least one year of work experience, a PT may volunteer to be or may be recruited as a CI. The PT may prepare for this teaching role (1) informally under the guidance of a CCCE, (2) through self-study. (3) through a series of more formal training sessions in the clinical center or affiliated physical therapy programs, or (4) through certification programs offered by the APTA and many of the regional consortiums of physical therapy educational programs.

CIs face the challenge of maintaining the quality of patient care and meeting productivity goals while providing learning experiences for students assigned to part-time or full-time extended internships. PTs seek the additional work and responsibility of a CI for a number of reasons: to "give back" to the profession out of gratitude to the CIs who taught them, share their expertise, remain current or to refresh skills and knowledge by teaching others, or modify their daily routines. CAPTE has established criteria for clinical faculty members[9] (Box 7-5).

In each center with a physical therapy clinical education program, one person is assigned the role of CCCE; this individual administers, manages, and coordinates the assignment of CIs and the clinical learning activities of students. The CCCE determines the readiness of PTs to serve as CIs and supervises their clinical teaching, discusses students' clinical performance with academic faculty members, and provides information about the center's clinical education programs to PT and PTA programs. Depending on the size of the center and the number of CIs, the CCCE's patient care and CI responsibilities may be reduced to allow time for CCCE duties; the position is considered supervisory or administrative. In smaller centers, the CI and CCCE may be the same person and the only one engaged in clinical education.

Box 7-5   **CRITERIA FOR CLINICAL PHYSICAL THERAPY FACULTY**[*]

2.2.5. The clinical education faculty demonstrates clinical expertise in their area of practice and the capacity to perform as effective clinical teachers.

The clinical education faculty are those clinicians who have the responsibility for education and supervision of students at clinical education sites. Members of the clinical education faculty serve as role models for students in scholarly and professional activities. Judgment about clinical education faculty competence is based on appropriate past and current involvement in in-service or continuing education courses; advanced degree courses; clinical experience; research experience; and teaching experience (e.g., classroom, clinical, in-service and/or continuing education). Clinical education faculty must have a minimum of 1 year of professional experience (2 years of clinical experience are preferred). Their continued ability to perform as clinical education faculty is assessed based on the individual's prior performance as a clinical educator and on other criteria established by the program.

From American Physical Therapy Association. Preface and introduction to the *CAPTE accreditation handbook 2002*. Retrieved November 9, 2003, at www.apta.org/Documents/Public/Accred/AppendixB-PT-Criteria.pdf. This material is copyrighted, and any further reproduction or distribution is prohibited.

[*]Criteria established by the Commission on Accreditation of Physical Therapy Education.

The CCCE is responsible for the quality of the clinical education program and for keeping current on issues such as billing for services provided by students, evaluation of student performance, and scheduling of students, who often are from several different PT and PTA programs. The CCCE plays an important role in integrating a clinical education program into the goals of a physical therapy organization. In an informal arrangement, a PT is asked to volunteer to serve as CI, which is perceived as extra duty, and student placement is unpredictable. When clinical education is tightly integrated into an organization's structure, students become part of the culture of the organization, and clinical instruction is an expected part of the job for every qualified PT.

One of the CCCE's responsibilities is overseeing reimbursement for student services under Medicare Part B[10] (Box 7-6). The rules governing such services reflect Medicare's concern that reimbursement be provided only for skilled physical therapy services; a PT, therefore, must be directly involved in the patient care for which Medicare is billed. State laws governing the practice of physical therapy also typically require that students be directly supervised. Such regulations pose a challenge to CIs, who must directly supervise students while gradually improving their ability to perform tasks independently.

The Clinical Performance Instrument (CPI), which was developed by the APTA as a means of evaluating student performance in clinical education, defines a student capable of entry-level practice as "a student who consistently and efficiently provides quality care with simple or complex patients and in a variety of clinical environments. The student usually needs no guidance or supervision except when addressing new or complex situations."[11] As the student progresses through the clinical education program under appropriate supervision and guidance, "the degree of monitoring or cueing needed is expected to progress from full-time monitoring or cueing for assistance to independent performance with consultation."[11]

Box 7-6   **MEDICARE PART B RULES FOR STUDENT PROVISION OF SERVICES**

The following are circumstances under which a provided service is considered provided directly by the practitioner and thus is billable, even though the student has some involvement in the patient's care:

- The qualified practitioner is recognized by the Medicare Part B beneficiary as the responsible professional in any session in which services are delivered.
- The qualified practitioner is present in the room for the entire session. The student participates in the delivery of services when the qualified practitioner is directing the service, making the skilled judgment, and is responsible for the assessment and treatment.
- The qualified practitioner is present in the room and guides the student in service delivery when the therapy student and the therapy assistant student are participating in the provision of services; the practitioner is not engaged in treating another patient or performing other tasks at the same time.
- The qualified practitioner is responsible for the services and therefore signs all documentation. (A student may also sign, but this is not necessary, because the Part B payment is made for the services of the clinician, not those of the student.)

Modified from Centers for Medicare and Medicaid Services. *Medicare carriers manual. Part 3: Claims process.* Transmittal 1753. Retrieved November 9, 2003, at http://www.hcfa.gov/pubforms/transmit/ R1753B3.pdf

Reconciling the reimbursement and legal demands for supervision of student performance with the instructional demand for independent performance is a major challenge for the clinical instructor.

The academic component of clinical education is the responsibility of the academic coordinator of clinical education (ACCE) or the director of clinical education (DCE)[12] (Box 7-7). These are atypical faculty positions because of the additional administrative duties. The ACCE role often serves as a stepping stone for clinical faculty members who want to move into an academic position.

Teaching Opportunities in Continuing Education

PTs are deluged with announcements of continuing education (nonacademic) courses, which traditionally are offered in seminars or during professional conferences and regional meetings. However, with the emergence of the computer and the Internet as educational tools, continuing education courses now can be offered as interactive web-based courses or home-based independent study programs that use texts or computer-delivered content.

Qualified PTs may take the initiative in sharing their expertise by offering a continuing education program, or they may be asked to volunteer to make presentations, particularly at regional professional programs. PTs may also choose to affiliate with a company in the continuing education business. In such cases the PT is paid to teach the course but is not responsible for the development, credentialing, or marketing aspects. Such arrangements can be lucrative for both parties, but restrictions may be imposed on presenters in terms of the content, frequency, and format of the courses.

Box 7-7   **RESPONSIBILITIES OF THE ACADEMIC COORDINATOR OF CLINICAL EDUCATION (ACCE) OR DIRECTOR OF CLINICAL EDUCATION (DCE)**

The ACCE/DCE holds a faculty (academic or clinical) appointment and has administrative, academic, service, and scholarship responsibilities consistent with the mission and philosophy of the academic program. In addition, the ACCE/DCE has primary responsibility for the following activities:

- Developing, monitoring, and refining the clinical education component of the curriculum
- Facilitating quality learning experiences for students during clinical education
- Evaluating students' performance, in cooperation with other faculty members, to determine the students' ability to integrate didactic and clinical learning experiences and to progress in the curriculum
- Educating students and clinical and academic faculty members about clinical education
- Selecting clinical learning environments that demonstrate the characteristics of sound patient/client management, ethical and professional behavior, and current physical therapy practice
- Maximizing available resources for the clinical education program
- Keeping records and providing assessments of the clinical education component (e.g., clinical education sites and clinical educators)
- Engaging core faculty members in clinical education planning, implementation, and assessment

---

From the American Physical Therapy Association. *Model position description for the academic coordinator/director of clinical education* (rev. 2002). Retrieved November 9, 2003, at http://www.apta.org/educatorinfo/model_position. This material is copyrighted, and any further reproduction or distribution is prohibited.

An entrepreneurial PT can create a continuing education program, although this requires skills beyond professional expertise. For each course offered, the following components must be addressed:

- Target audience and marketing plan
- Clearly defined rationale and learning objectives
- Learning outcomes
- Instructional strategies
- Presentation format (seminar, distance learning, home study)
- Audiovisual or other technological expertise required to present content
- Length of course
- Determination of continuing education units to be awarded
- Approval of the course by the appropriate credentialing organization
- Plan for documentation of attendance and filing of permanent records
- Fee for the course based on expenses and profit
- Course evaluation method

Continuing education is a market-driven industry that presents entrepreneurial opportunities as well as sources of revenue for professional associations. National criteria have been established for colleges, associations, and companies that wish to be credentialed to award *continuing education units (CEUs)*, the standard time increments for measuring the value of continuing education courses.[13] Approval of a course by one of these organizations gives some assurance that the instructors are qualified to present the course and that the learning objectives are reasonable.

Although the credentialing process is a step in the right direction, concern still exists about the quality of course content and the evidence supporting the content. For example, those assigned to review courses for CEUs may not be content experts. Also, the information presented may be based on personal experience rather than scientific evidence; this perpetuates the lack of evidence-based physical therapy tests and interventions, particularly if the course involves the presentation of new treatment strategies. These issues cloud the CEU requirement for licensure renewal. Whether accumulation of a required number of CEUs truly reflects a PT's efforts to maintain or improve clinical competence is unclear, and the professions must depend on the market to determine the popularity and acceptance of continuing education programs.

Academic Teaching Opportunities

PTs may maintain their clinical practice and serve as guest lecturers in physical therapy and PTA programs. Some type of honorarium may be offered, but more often these are unpaid teaching opportunities rewarded with letters of appreciation. However, serving as guest lecturers allows PTs to explore their interest and skills in classroom teaching. Also, guest lecturers may be treated less formally than full-time academic instructors; they may not have to submit detailed credentials or allow evaluative review of assignments by administrators. Faculty members assigned to courses identify those in the community with expertise that complements or supplements the course content and invite them to take part in classroom instruction. The guest lecturer may participate in a single course or may present the same topic each time the course is offered.

The most formal teaching opportunity for PTs is a position as a full-time or part-time (adjunct) faculty member in a PT or PTA curriculum. Faculty positions are based on the academic triad of teaching, research, and service. The distribution of the faculty's efforts among these three elements, as well as the performance expectations for faculty members, vary according to the type of institution (e.g., private or public, research or liberal arts) and the availability of tenure. For example, in community colleges, the emphasis is on teaching, with very little expectation of faculty research. In large universities, the expectations for research (production and dissemination of new knowledge) and for obtaining external funding to support the research tend to overshadow efforts in the other areas. In smaller colleges, the focus may be more on teaching responsibilities and publication of new information. Cutting across these institutional differences, CAPTE[14] has clarified the scholarship expectations for each faculty member in a physical therapy program, which are based on Boyer's categories of scholarship—discovery, integration, application, and teaching[15]:

- *Scholarship of discovery* focuses on the development or creation of new knowledge by traditional research that is disseminated through peer-reviewed publications and through professional presentation of grants awarded for research or theory development, recognition of scholarship, and outcome studies.
- *Scholarship of integration* involves critical analysis and review of knowledge within disciplines and creative insights derived from different disciplines or fields of study. Such work may involve publication of literature reviews, meta-analyses, and synthesis of the literature from other disciplines accompanied by discussion of its significance for physical therapy. This form of scholarship also includes the publication of books and book chapters, reports on service projects, and policy presentations designed to influence the positions of professional organizations and government agencies.
- *Scholarship of application* is the use of knowledge to solve real problems in the professions, industry, government, and the community. The findings obtained through scholarship of discovery and scholarship of integration are applied to clinical practice or teaching and learning. This process may result in consultation reports, products, licenses, copyrights, and grants supporting innovations in practice.
- *Scholarship of teaching* involves critical reflection on and dissemination of knowledge about teaching and learning. It includes classroom assessment and evidence gathering, the use of contemporary teaching theories applicable to the particular profession, peer collaboration and review, and inquiry into issues related to student learning. Scholarship of teaching is not synonymous simply with excellent teaching; it also requires the individual to produce published, peer-reviewed articles devoted to pedagogy, to devise teaching innovations, to merit recognition as a master teacher, to write textbooks on teaching, and to obtain grants and make presentations related to issues in teaching and learning.

CAPTE differentiates service responsibilities as *internal service* (e.g., serving on departmental and college committees) and *external service* (e.g., holding elected office in professional organizations or serving on boards of community organizations).

To meet the institutional and CAPTE criteria for a faculty appointment, the PT must pursue or have completed graduate study (the doctoral degree is heavily preferred in physical therapy education) and must be comfortable to some degree with moving away from direct patient care. The transition to faculty member from clinical practice may be difficult, because the responsibilities are quite different and often surprising. The transition may startle even individuals who have had peripheral contact with the academic world as guest lecturers, because faculty members' responsibilities extend far beyond preparation of a lecture or course and the duties of the teaching-research-service triad. Faculty members also develop curricula and courses, prepare syllabi, choose instructional strategies, evaluate student performance, and contribute to the student admission process. This involvement of the entire faculty in collegial decision making to meet the needs of professional education is very different from clinical working relationships.

THEORIES OF TEACHING AND LEARNING IN PROFESSIONAL EDUCATION

Regardless of the audience, the effectiveness of teaching is determined to some degree by how well the teacher understands the ways in which people learn (Table 7-1).

A teacher's philosophy of learning directs instructional strategy. Purists contend that effectiveness may be compromised if learning theories are mixed; others strongly believe that an eclectic approach is critical when a wide range of information and skills must be learned. For example, knowledge acquisition can be achieved in a variety of ways. Initial knowledge acquisition is perhaps best served by the classical instruction method, with predetermined learning outcomes, sequenced instructional interaction, and criterion-referenced evaluation. Patient problem solving and integration of information, on the other hand, may be better taught from an andragogic perspective (see Table 7-1).

An important tool from the behaviorist approach that is useful for all instruction is a taxonomy of educational objectives, based on the early work of Benjamin Bloom (Box 7-8). Learning behaviors are classified into three domains: the cognitive domain (recall and use of information), the psychomotor domain (physical and manipulative skills), and the affective domain (interest, attitudes, and values). In each domain, learning is organized into a hierarchy of complexity. In the cognitive domain, for example, analysis of information is a much higher learning objective than recall of knowledge. This taxonomy is helpful for determining the level of learning expected, and it provides the verbs for writing objectives.

In devising a teaching plan, whether for a group, an in-service presentation, or a graduate course, the instructor should begin with the purpose or expected outcome (or outcomes) of the learning unit. The outcomes should be classified according to the taxonomy described previously so that objectives in specific terminal behaviors, or the outcomes of the learning that the student must demonstrate, can be developed. Examples of terminal behaviors are found in Box 7-9 in the "B" part of each learning objective. The instructional method and the evaluation tool most appropriate for each domain can then be identified. For example, if psychomotor goals are sought, laboratory practice is indicated, and a practical examination would be the test of choice. With affective goals, discussion groups and a report may be indicated.

ETHICAL AND LEGAL ISSUES IN PHYSICAL THERAPY EDUCATION

Teachers are also responsible for understanding ethical and legal issues. A sample of education legislation is presented in Table 7-2 to reflect the complexity of the higher education process. Discrimination, privacy, dismissal policies, and academic freedom are among the issues.

Table 7-1 | **Learning Theories**

	Behaviorism	Cognitivism	Constructivism	Andragogy
Theorists	Aristotle, Hobbs, Pavlov, Watson, Thorndike, Skinner	Tolman, Bandura	Bartlett, Bruner, Piaget, Kant, Kuhn, Dewey and Habermas	Knowles
Principles	The theory concentrates on the study of overt behaviors that can be observed and measured; the mind is viewed as a "black box." Stimulus-response can be observed quantitatively, and feedback is a motivator. The possibility of thought processes occurring in the mind is ignored, and the theory does not explain social behavior.	The individual can model behavior by observing the behavior of another person. Learning involves associations established through contiguity and repetition, and reinforcement provides feedback on correct responses. Learning involves acquisition or reorganization of the cognitive structures through which humans process and store information. Cognitive scientists believe humans process information in a manner similar to that of computers: receive, store, and retrieve	Learners construct (interpret) their own reality based on their perceptions of experiences. Knowledge is a function of one's prior experiences, mental structures, and beliefs, which are used to interpret objects and events. Humans perceive pretty much the same way, and reality is shared through a process of social negotiation.	This theory applies specifically to adult learning. Adults are self-directed and expect to take responsibility for decisions. The following assumptions are made about the design of learning: (1) Adults need to know why they need to learn something; (2) adults need to learn experientially; (3) adults approach learning as problem solving; (4) adults learn best when the topic is of immediate value; (5) adults must be willing to learn the subject matter (i.e., readiness to learn).
Strengths	Learner focuses on a clear goal and can respond automatically to the cues of that goal.	All learners are trained to do a task the same way to ensure consistency.	Learners are able to interpret multiple realities and better able to deal with real-life situations. If learners can problem solve,	Learners focus on the process and develop as problem solvers; that is, they imitate real life.

Continued

Table 7-1 | Learning Theories—cont'd

	Behaviorism	Cognitivism	Constructivism	Andragogy
Weaknesses	In some situations the stimulus for the correct response does not occur; therefore the learners cannot respond because they do not understand the system.	Learners are taught a way to accomplish a task, but it may not be the best way, or it may not be suited to the learner or the situation.	they may better apply their existing knowledge to a new situation. In situations in which conformity is essential, divergent thinking and action may cause problems.	The focus is on the process rather than specific content; more than one correct answer may exist. Evaluation of performance may be difficult.
Suitable uses in teaching	Tasks or information that requires little processing (e.g., basic paired associations, discriminations, rote memorization).	Tasks requiring a higher level of processing (e.g., classifications), rule making or procedural executions that have a stronger cognitive emphasis (e.g., schematic organization, analogical reasoning, algorithmic problem solving).	Tasks demanding high levels of processing (e.g., experimental problem solving, personal selection and monitoring of cognitive strategies).	Adults or any age group when the task is student focused.
Instructional strategies	Behavioral objectives movement, teaching machine, programmed instruction, computer-assisted instruction.	Use of advance organizers, mnemonic devices, metaphors, chunking into meaningful parts, and careful organization of instructional materials from simple to complex.	Situated learning, cognitive apprenticeships, social negotiation; use of hypertext and hypermedia, which allow for a branched design instead of a linear instructional format. Hyperlinks allow learner control, which is crucial to constructivists.	Case studies, role playing, simulations, problem-based learning, and self-evaluation. Instructors adopt the role of facilitator or resource rather than lecturer or grader.

Modified from Merria SB, Caffarella RS. Learning in adulthood. A comprehensive guide. San Francisco: Jossey-Bass, 1998.

Box 7-8   TAXONOMY OF LEARNING OBJECTIVES

Cognitive Domain	Psychomotor Domain	Affective Domain
Knowledge	*Perception*	*Receiving*
Recall	Awareness via sense organs	Perception of a stimulus
Comprehension	*Set*	*Responding*
Purposeful organization	Readiness for action	Reaction to the stimulus
Application	*Guided response*	*Valuing*
Concrete use of abstractions	Tutored behavior	Commitment to the stimulus
Analysis	*Mechanism*	*Organization*
Expression of relationships among ideas	Habit	Formation of a value system
Synthesis	*Complex overt response*	*Ideals*
Combination of ideas to form new concepts	Series of coordinated motor skills	Formation of a total philosophy
Evaluation		
Formation of judgments		

Modified from Bemis KA, Schroeder GB. *Writing and use of behavioral objectives*. Albuquerque, NM: Southwestern Cooperative Education Lab; 1969. ED033881.

Box 7-9   ABCD METHOD OF WRITING LEARNING OBJECTIVES

Each learning objective has four parts:
A—Audience (Who is the learner?)
B—Behavior (What will the learner be expected to do?)
C—Condition (What are the conditions of the action?)
D—Degree (How often will it be done?)

Sample Learning Objectives
Cognitive domain
The student (A) will analyze the components of a postsurgical aquatic exercise program (B) for an individual who has undergone repair of the rotator cuff (C). The student will apply Archimedes' principles with occasional cues from the instructor (D).

Psychomotor domain
The student (A) will conduct a postsurgical aquatic exercise (B) for a patient who has undergone repair of the rotator cuff (C) independently (D).

Affective domain
The student (A) will discuss the comparative value of postsurgical aquatic exercises (B) for a patient who has undergone repair of the rotator cuff (C), using a variety of perspectives with no prompts for inclusion of possible alternatives (D).

Modified from Mager RF. *Preparing instructional objectives* (3rd ed). Atlanta: Center for Effective Performance; 1997.

Table 7-2 | **Selected Legislation and Case Law Affecting Higher Education**

Title	Purpose	Information Source
Family Educational Rights and Privacy Act (1974)	Protects the privacy of student records	www.ed.gov/offices/OM/fpco/ferpa/
Section 504 and Title II of the Americans with Disabilities Act (1973)	Prevents discrimination based on disability	www.ed.gov/offices/OCR/disability.html
Keyishian v. Board of Regents, 385 U.S. 589 (1967)	Ensures academic freedom	www.clhe.org/academicfreedom/page1.shtml
University of California Berkeley Regents v. Bakke, 438 U.S. 265 (1978)	Supports affirmative action	www.clhe.org/affirmativeaction/page1.shtml
Title IX Education Amendments of 1972 (1972)	Forbids discrimination based on gender in programs and activities	www.clhe.org/studentaffairs/page1.shtml
University of Missouri v. Horowitz, 435 U.S. 90 (1978)	Addresses dismissal of students for noncognitive (behavioral or clinical) performance	www.law.umkc.edu/faculty/projects/ftrials/conlaw/horowitz.html
McDonald v. Hogness, 92 Wn.2d431, at 437 (1979)	Prohibits arbitrary and capricious decisions on student performance	www.mrss.org/mc/courts/supreme/092win2d/092win2d0431.htm

APTA Code of Ethics and *Guide for Professional Conduct*

Principle 6 of the APTA *Code of Ethics* obligates physical therapists to "maintain and promote high standards for physical therapy practice, education, and research."[16] The association's *Guide for Profession Conduct*[17] (GPC) elaborates on this principle, linking it to continual self-assessment to determine compliance with professional standards (GPC 6.1), professional competence and quality improvement (GPC 6.2), support for high-quality professional education (GPC 6.3), continuing education (GPC 6.4), and support for research (GPC 6.5). The ethical obligations of PTs involved in teaching or continuing education are specifically addressed. PTs providing continuing education courses should be competent in the content (GPC 6.4A) and should give accurate information about the course in course materials (GPC 6.4B).[17] Those attending continuing education courses are obligated to evaluate the quality of the information before putting it to use: "A physical therapist shall evaluate the efficacy and effectiveness of information and techniques presented in continuing education programs before integrating them into his/her practice" (GPC 6.4C).[17]

Continuing Competence

The quality of continuing education and its contribution to continuing competence are issues of particular concern to state practice boards, which are charged with protecting the public from professional incompetence. By granting a license, the licensing board signifies that it has determined the PT is competent to practice. As stated by the APTA *Code of Ethics* and *Guide for Professional Conduct*, maintaining competence requires commitment to a lifelong process of education and skill development to meet the ever-changing needs of health care. Mandatory continuing education has been the tool most commonly used to ensure that licensed PTs maintain competence, although it is universally acknowledged that attendance at courses does not necessarily translate into competence. The Federation of State Boards of Physical Therapy has established standards of continuing competence for physical therapy and has committed itself to developing measurement tools for assessing competence.[18]

Academic Integrity

Programs that educate future professionals seemingly would be free of cheating and violations of academic integrity; however, educational journals indicate that this is not the case. Technology has created additional challenges to academic integrity by making materials easier to copy. Also, students have been caught sending messages by cell phone during practical examinations. As with any type of cheating, sanctions for such actions must balance the ultimate good of the student against the responsibilities of the educational and gatekeeping roles. Because self-regulation is expected of professionals, serious violations of academic integrity may be considered an indication that a student lacks the required moral qualities and decision-making capability.

Vulnerability of Students

Just as patients are vulnerable to the PT's knowledge and status, students are vulnerable to the status and power of faculty members. Students may be subjected to unfair grading, sexual harassment, or discrimination. Clinical faculty members have particular power over students because the faculty members may make judgments that are somewhat subjective without direct input from academic faculty members. A study of covert bias among 83 physical therapists found that the PTs gave black students lower ratings on a presentation than they did white and Asian students, even though the presentations were identical in content.[19] The results of the study are disturbing in light of the small number of minorities in physical therapy. Furthermore, academic educators may be reluctant to challenge clinical faculty members for fear of losing scarce clinical placement sites.

ETHICS LITERATURE AND THE EDUCATOR'S ROLE

From 1970 to 2000, significantly fewer articles in the ethics literature addressed issues arising from the PT's role as educator (9.9%) than addressed issues involved in the patient/client management role (48.1%) (see Figure 4-5). Most of the articles on the educator's role dealt with the structure and content of the physical therapy ethics curriculum.[20]

SUMMARY

Teaching roles for PTs range from one-on-one patient/client management to full-time teaching with little or no patient care. The PT educator may have an informal preparation or may have completed graduate studies in education. The transition from clinician to full-time educator involves career planning, because academic positions require advanced degrees.

PTs who want to pursue professional development by obtaining an academic position should consider the following factors:
- Their level of self-confidence as an expert in some area of physical therapy
- Their level of comfort with public speaking
- Their commitment to research and service as well as teaching
- The importance of effective teaching and learning strategies
- The complicated milieu of higher education and the responsibility inherent in the preparation of licensed professionals

Community colleges, continuing education courses, and technological advances that support nontraditional methods of instruction also provide teaching opportunities beyond the traditional professional programs. The complexity of the educator's role at all these levels is reflected in the legal and ethical challenges that must be met. The following scenarios provide opportunities to explore the role of the PT as educator.

CASE SCENARIOS

Case Scenario 1

The physical therapy staff of Riverfront Health Care Systems contributes to the hospital's community education series. You have been asked to participate in the new "My Baby and Me" program. The target audience is pregnant women in their last trimester who will continue with the class for 3 months after giving birth. The goal of the program is to improve the health of pregnant women and their babies before and after birth. New groups will be formed the first of every month, and the groups will meet every other week. You are to determine the subject matter you would like to teach, the number of 1-hour sessions needed to complete the program, and the resources required. Guest speakers will include nurses, physicians, social workers, and psychologists.
- *Prepare a memo that provides the information requested, as well as learning goals for the program.*

Case Scenario 2

You have been on the staff of the Gentle Care Skilled Nursing Home for about 2 years. You are the only PT who supervises two PTAs. All-State University, which is in the same city, has asked you to consider an affiliation agreement to offer educational opportunities for students in the second year of physical therapy school. Although you have held other positions, you have never served as a clinical instructor.
- *What questions should you ask before deciding whether to become a clinical instructor?*

Case Scenario 3

Because of the reputation your practice has achieved in the rehabilitation of individuals with multiple sclerosis, you and two other PTs have been approached by Professional

Education, Inc., a provider of continuing education courses for rehabilitation professionals, to develop an 8-hour rehabilitation course for people with multiple sclerosis. Assume that you and your colleagues have accepted the offer and are satisfied with the financial arrangements.

- *What steps do you take to develop the course?*

Case Scenario 4

All-State University has asked you to present a lecture on the challenges facing pediatric PTs who provide services in public school systems. You have 30 minutes and are expected to use slides.

- *Prepare your presentation, including the slides.*

Case Scenario 5

You have been appointed to a new task force in your chapter of the APTA. The group is charged with advising the Board of Physical Therapy Practice in your state in the development of policies that would establish continuing education requirements as proof of continuing or improved competency for licensed PTs and PTAs.

- *What are your preliminary thoughts as you prepare for the first meeting of the task force?*

Case Scenario 6

You have served as a clinical instructor for students from All-State University for 6 years. During a conversation with a student, the individual inadvertently reveals that she and two classmates routinely have cheated on examinations while in physical therapy school. When you express your surprise, she replies that it is common knowledge that "everyone cheats"—otherwise students could never manage all the courses and studying required by physical therapy. The student asks you not to discuss the matter with faculty members at the university because, if word gets out about her slip of the lip, other students will never forgive her.

- *What do you do?*

REFERENCES

1. American Physical Therapy Association. *The interactive guide to physical therapist practice with catalog of tests and measures* (version 1.0). Alexandria, Va: The Association; 2002.
2. McMillan M. *Massage and therapeutic exercise*, 3rd ed. Philadelphia: WB Saunders; 1932.
3. American Physical Therapy Association. *The beginnings: Physical therapy and the APTA*. Alexandria, Va: The Association; 1979.
4. Murphy W. *Healing the generations: A history of physical therapy and the American Physical Therapy Association*. Alexandria, Va: The Association; 1995.
5. American Physical Therapy Association. Commission on Accreditation in Physical Therapy Education, 2004 fact sheets for PT and PTA programs. Retrieved November 9, 2003, at http://www.apta.org/education/accreditation/fact_sheets
6. American Physical Therapy Association. *A normative model of physical therapist professional education: Version 2000*. Alexandria, Va: The Association; 2001.
7. American Physical Therapy Association. *APTA vision statement*. Retrieved November 9, 2003, at http://www.apta.org/About/aptamissiongoals/visionstatement
8. Churchill RE. Information management in public health settings [course]. Tampa, Fla:University of South Florida College of Public Health; summer 2001.

9. American Physical Therapy Association. Preface and introduction to the CAPTE accreditation handbook 2002. Retrieved November 9, 2003, at http://www.apta.org/Education/accreditation/accreditation_handbook

10. Centers for Medicare and Medicaid Services. Medicare carriers manual. Part 3: Claims process. Transmittal 1753. Retrieved November 9, 2003, at http://www.hcfa.gov/pubforms/transmit/R1753B3.pdf

11. American Physical Therapy Association. *Physical therapist clinical performance instrument*. Alexandria, Va: The Association; 1997.

12. American Physical Therapy Association. *Model position description for the academic coordinator/director of clinical education (rev. 2002)*. Retrieved November 9, 2003, at http://www.apta.org/Education/educatorinfo/model_position

13. International Association for Continuing Education and Training. *Proven standards for quality in continuing education and training*. Retrieved November 9, 2003, http://at www.iacet.org/about/ceu.htm

14. American Physical Therapy Association. *White paper on scholarship in the position papers adopted by CAPTE*. Retrieved November 9, 2003, at http://www.apta.org/pdfs/accreditation/AppendixE-POSITION-PAPERS-ADOPTED-BY-CAPTE.pdf

15. Boyer EL. *Scholarship reconsidered*. San Francisco: Jossey-Bass; 1997.

16. American Physical Therapy Association. *APTA code of ethics*. Retrieved October 27, 2004, at http://www.apta.org/AM/Template.cfm?

17. American Physical Therapy Association. *APTA guide for professional conduct*. Retrieved October 27, 2004, at http://www.apta.org/AM/Template.cfm?

18. Federation of State Boards of Physical Therapy. *Standards of competence* (approved by the board of directors, August, 2000). Retrieved November 9, 2003, at http://www.fsbpt.org/standards.htm

19. Haskins AR, Rose-St Prix C, Elbaum L. Covert bias in evaluation of physical therapist students' clinical performance. *Phys Ther* 1997;77:155-168.

20. Swisher LL. A retrospective analysis of ethics knowledge in physical therapy (1970-2000). *Phys Ther* 2002;82:592-706.

8

The Physical Therapist as Administrator

Administration is the skilled process of planning, directing, organizing, and managing human, technical, environmental, and financial resources effectively and efficiently. Administration includes the management, by individual physical therapists, of resources for patient/client management and for organizational operations.

– The Interactive Guide to Physical Therapist Practice with Catalog of Tests and Measures version 1.0 (2002)[1]

THE HISTORY OF PHYSICAL THERAPY ADMINISTRATION

Physical therapists (PTs) have been administrators from the very beginning of the profession. As chief aides, PTs supervised other reconstruction aides in the treatment of wounded soldiers returning from World War I, and they subsequently worked with orthopedists as equal partners to provide rehabilitation services for civilian patients. After World War II, physical medicine and rehabilitation emerged as a medical specialty. Physician specialists in this field, called *physiatrists*, were responsible for the overall management of rehabilitation units in hospitals, and in the military tradition, each discipline of the rehabilitation department had a "chief" (e.g., chief PT, chief occupational therapist).

Because a high percentage of PTs were employed by hospitals, a typical career pattern for a staff PT involved promotion to a supervisory position; this typically meant the PT assumed responsibility for training and assigning the duties of support personnel and perhaps some responsibility for scheduling staff and patients for a particular subunit, such as outpatient services. The next step up the career ladder was the administrative "chief" position, which involved hiring, evaluating, and firing staff members; purchasing supplies and equipment; and collaborating with other members of the rehabilitation and health care teams. However, PTs had very little opportunity for advancement to such administrative positions in this physician-dominated, hospital-based, bureaucratic model, which also characterized community-based organizations such as the Easter Seal Society and other groups that provided services to children and adults with chronic conditions.

As an employment alternative, PTs could work directly with a physician (typically an orthopedist or a physiatrist), providing services in the physician's office. These positions also involved some administrative functions, depending on the number of people providing physical therapy services and the extent to which the physician delegated management of the practice to the PT.

Just as the health care system has changed over the past decades, so has the management of physical therapy services. Beginning in the 1960s, physicians were increasingly replaced as managers of hospital rehabilitation services by professional health care managers, who were academically prepared to deal with the increasing complexity of health care delivery. Some of these new, midlevel managers were PTs and other health care professionals who had acquired management skills through graduate studies or work experience. Others, who were not health care professionals, had business degrees that focused on health care. This insertion of business practices and overseers who are not health professionals into the management of health care may be either a cause or a result (or perhaps both) of health care becoming an industry rather than a service.

In the late 1960s, more entrepreneurial PTs began developing independent private practices, and for-profit corporations were formed to provide outpatient rehabilitation services in numerous centers, often nationwide. Freestanding private physical therapy practices became commonplace. The provision of skilled services in nursing homes offered new opportunities for these PTs as Medicare reimbursement for rehabilitation services in skilled nursing homes became lucrative. In addition to providing direct patient care services in freestanding clinics, PTs created companies through which they contracted their services to health care organizations.

For health care organizations, outsourcing physical therapy services to rehabilitation companies has several advantages, including the following:

- Reducing direct costs and providing flexibility in coping with periods of change
- Freeing up more time for focusing on organizational tasks rather than supervision of staff
- Allowing access to a critical mass of expertise not available in-house

For PTs, outsourcing may be a means of enhancing professional autonomy in a variety of work settings, increasing flexibility in the amount and scheduling of work, and benefiting from the ability to focus on a particular specialty for career development.[2]

These incentives are more attractive to independent contractors than to PTs who work for physical therapy contracting organizations, essentially as employees. However, PTs in the latter situation at least work for other PTs, who are more likely to have significant insight into important professional and clinical issues.

Outsourcing has two important disadvantages, which have the greatest impact when the need for physical therapy services is unpredictable. First, PTs run the risk of income loss for uncertain periods of time. Second, PTs may be unavailable when, from the manager's perspective, they are most needed by the health care organization.

PTs also practice in public school systems. The school system may employ the PTs directly, or it may contract out physical therapy services to individual PTs or other organizations. PTs in school systems often provide services at several schools and work closely with teachers and other therapists to establish goals for each student's individualized education plan.

Another model of practice recently has emerged. A corporation provides an umbrella for outpatient physical therapy centers which provide support for PTs who independently manage their own practices. This arrangement has the potential to provide the best of both worlds for a PT: the PT enjoys a great deal of autonomy in the day-to-day management of a practice but has the business support needed for developing the practice, marketing, billing, and other financial responsibilities.

In health care systems, the recent trend has been to move away from discipline-specific departments toward program, or product-line management. For example, instead of the traditional physical therapy, occupational therapy, speech and language pathology, and nursing departments, a hospital or medical center now may be organized into patient-centered programs or units, such as the orthopedic service, the stroke center, or the head trauma unit. This model has several advantages: the team of professionals assigned to the program develops an expertise with patients who have a particular diagnosis, and teamwork becomes easier, resulting in greater efficiency in communication and treatment. The managers of these units typically come from one of the participating disciplines, so a PT may be managed by a nurse or occupational therapist or may supervise professionals from a variety of disciplines.

Despite these advantages, the program model raises concerns about professional identity and autonomy that are similar to those that arise when the manager of the service is a professional manager with no credentials in a health care discipline or when physicians manage rehabilitation services.

All employment situations pose the threat of loss of professional autonomy. Mark[2] suggests that employed PTs may have less professional accountability and a diminished guarantee of maintaining professional expertise because they must rely on managers who are not physical therapy professionals for access to training and development. Also, employed PTs may have less professional interaction with other PTs and much less flexibility to provide or receive cover from PTs working in competing areas of the organization.[2]

CONTEMPORARY PHYSICAL THERAPY ADMINISTRATION

Physical therapists now have many more opportunities to assume managerial responsibility in a wider range of organizational structures at different levels of management. The development of skills for managerial roles is more important than ever, and even without an administrative or a managerial title, PTs arguably call upon many of these skills in providing direct patient care.

Because no theory of administration exists per se and because the terms *administration* and *management* often are used interchangeably, the role of first-level manager, often considered an administrative position, is best understood from the broad base of management theory. (The term *manager* is used interchangeably with *administrator* for this purpose.)

Management is the process by which an organization meets its goals. Managers are responsible for selecting the procedures to be used and for evaluating the effectiveness and efficiency of these procedures in meeting the stated goals. The arrangement of the management system depends on the size and complexity of the organization and the number of management levels.

Management theories, which originated in the early 20th century and have evolved since then, are closely related to organizational and leadership theories (Table 8-1). Organizations reflect a wide range and mix of these theories. Some remain strongly bureaucratic, with a definite chain of command. Others have a

Table 8-1 | Summary of Theories of Organization, Management, and Leadership

Time Period	Organization	Management	Leadership	Effect on Physical Therapy
Early 1900s	Industrial model; hierarchical, produced bureaucracies that still exist.	Classical management style; bureaucratic, based on time-motion studies and "one best way" theory (Weber, Taylor, Fayol, Follett).	Great man theory: Innate ability, born to lead; impresses will to induce obedience, respect, loyalty, cooperation.	Physical therapy not yet an organized discipline.
1920 to 1930	See early 1900s.	Human relations theory; worker attitudes affect productivity: zone of indifference concept developed—range in which willing to accept orders without question (Hawthorne, Barnard).	Group theory: Leadership emerges from a group through command-and-dominate; course of action of many is changed by one person.	Need for reconstruction aides to treat military wounded results in development of physical therapists (PTs) to meet civilian needs. PTs work under direction of orthopedists in their private practices or in hospitals.
1940 to 1950	See early 1900s.	Systems theory; organization is system of interrelated and interdependent parts functioning as a whole to accomplish a goal that one part alone cannot (Katz and Kahn).	Some traits are common to all leaders; the ability to persuade or direct does not depend on a title; followers lift a person to leadership.	Hospital-based physical therapy continues to be managed by physicians; PTs continue to work in physician practices.
1950 to 1960	See early 1900s.	Human resources theory; focus on motivation and leadership (Blake and Mouton).	Behavior theory: Key behavioral patterns result in leadership (e.g., ability to influence others to get a job done or to move a group toward goals).	Move is made toward PTs playing greater role in management.
1960 to 1970	See early 1900s.	Contingency theory; fit of organization processes to the characteristics of each situation. Applies other models as the situation dictates (Fiedler).	Contingency/situational theory: Certain behaviors succeed in certain situations. Includes a political perspective in that the inequality of influence guides collective behavior. Contingency leadership is the process of influencing others	Private practice, rehabilitation corporations develop; fewer PTs are hospital based. Professional managers replace discipline professionals as overseers.

	Business practices	Management theory	Leadership	Physical therapy
Early to late 1980s	Participative model emerges in which businesses are product based and use work teams to accomplish their goals.	Quality management theory; Structured system for satisfying customers through the integration of continuous improvement processes (Deming).	to perform beyond the expectations of those in authority. Leadership is the process of influencing others to perform beyond the expectations of those in authority. Role of organization's leadership is to promote a quest for excellence.	Rehabilitation corporations begin to emerge.
Late 1980s through 1990s	Business practices are marked by reengineering, downsizing, outsourcing, and multitasking.	Mixed management style; participative but management exerts more control. Transformational (Burns; Bennis and Nanus).	Leaders infuse values and purpose in an organization. Service leadership. Emergence of leadership "gurus."	Umbrella rehabilitation corporations that provide more independence in small practices emerge.
2000 and beyond	Globalization of labor market; diversity produces both innovation and conflict. Business practices marked by continued outsourcing and downsizing, strategic alliances with competitors and collaborators, customization, and decentralization.	Flexible management; customized employment with focus on lifetime employability rather than marked lifetime employment. Fewer levels of management, workers empowered to make decisions, fewer differences in responsibilities across layers, fewer policies and procedures. Aspects of participative model (Vroom and Yetton).	Networking allows direct communication, reducing the need for a chain of command across unit teams.	More PTs practice as independent contractors.

more flexible structure and management style that allow them to respond more easily to changes in missions and goals and permits greater employee participation at all levels in decisions about the organization.

As a professional trade organization that represents PTs and physical therapist assistants (PTAs), the American Physical Therapy Association (APTA) represents one type of organizational structure (Figure 8-1). The business of the membership is conducted through an elected body of representatives, the House of Delegates.[3] The executive committee of the board of directors oversees the headquarters' staff (Figure 8-2), which accomplishes the work of the association.[4]

The APTA appears to be very much a traditional, bureaucratic, hierarchical organization with a clear chain of command and very little connection among its five divisions (i.e., communication, education, finance and administration, governance/components/meetings, and practice/research). Even the designations used (e.g., *headquarters* and *divisions*) are military terms that suggest the underlying organizational and managerial model. In this type of organization, each division is responsible for a portion of the work "pie," and the work would be divided up into particular tasks. Each division head has the opportunity to meet regularly with all other division heads, probably in meetings chaired by the chief executive officer (CEO), but little day-to-day interaction occurs among the divisions to accomplish the goals of the organization. (See Case Scenario 1 for an opportunity to change the organizational structure of the APTA.)

Given the wide range of perspectives and to avoid bias toward any particular theory, physical therapy management is considered in this discussion on the basis of the responsibilities managers hold in four broad areas: finances, human resources, operations, and information (Table 8-2). Selected responsibilities that represent contemporary professional issues also are presented.

Another perspective on the division of managerial responsibilities focuses on the control an individual has at each management level over (1) work to be performed immediately, (2) future work, (3) the work of others, (4) the organization's goals, and (5) interaction with others at the same organizational level (Table 8-3).

Although managers at every level of a physical therapy organization have the same types of responsibility, the actual responsibilities vary. For discussion purposes, responsibilities are presented as exclusive to each management level; however, depending on the organization's structure and management style, some variation or overlap of responsibilities and titles may exist at adjacent levels. For example, a first-line manager may also have a full caseload of patients, or a staff PT may be assigned quality assurance duties.

PATIENT/CLIENT MANAGEMENT

The management of patients is the common level of management or administration for all PTs. In day-to-day patient/client management, PTs take charge of resources, plan the care of patients, direct support personnel, and organize time and work. Through these duties, the PT becomes a manager of the assigned work, responsible for ensuring that the outcomes of the care provided contribute to the organization's overall goals. Professional issues at this level of management include billing, documentation, and delegation and supervision of support personnel.

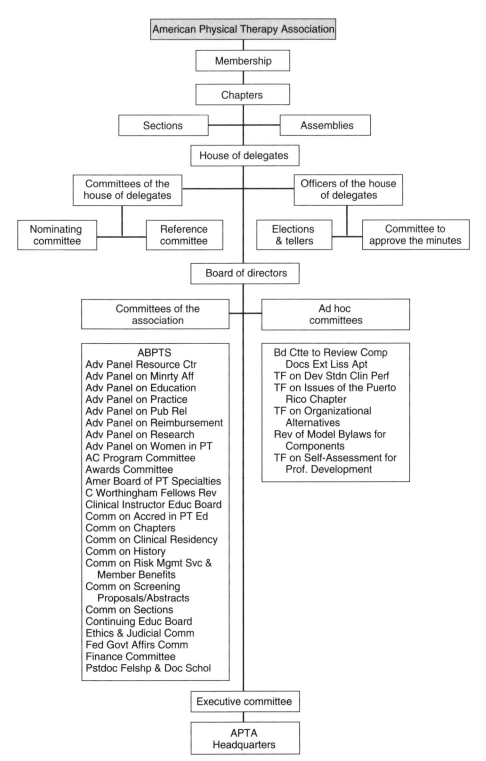

Figure 8-1. Organizational chart for the American Physical Therapy Association. *(From American Physical Therapy Association. APTA organizational chart. Retrieved November 9, 2003, at http://www.apta.org/AM/Template.cfm?Section=Search&section=Governance&template=/CM/ContentDisplay.cfm&ContentFileID=2698. This material is copyrighted, and any further reproduction distribution is prohibited.)*

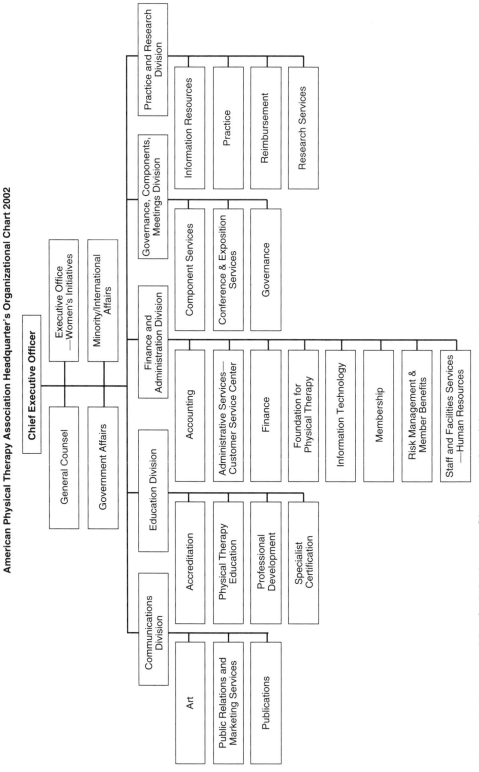

Figure 8-2. Organizational chart for the headquarters of the American Physical Therapy Association. *(From American Physical Therapy Association. APTA headquarters organization chart 2002. Retrieved November 9, 2003, at http://www.apta.org/AM/Template.cfm?Section=Search&section=Governance&template=/CM/ContentDisplay.cfm&ContentFileID=2699. This material is copyrighted and any further reproduction or distribution is prohibited.)*

Table 8-2 | **Levels of Management and Responsibilities in Physical Therapy**

Level of Management	Financial Responsibilities	Human Resources Responsibilities	Operations Responsibilities	Information Responsibilities
Patient/client patient management (i.e., staff physical therapist)	Oversees billing for services provided	Directs support personnel to implement parts of care plans	Schedules caseload; reports need for expendable supplies	Collects data; documents care
First-line manager (e.g., supervisor, administrator)	Monitors and reports revenue and expenses in budgeting process; requests funding and projects revenue	Hires and dismisses staff members and evaluates their performance; assigns staff to patients	Analyzes productivity; implements risk management program	Compiles and analyzes data for quality assurance and other internal reports
Mid-level manager (e.g., director, vice president)	Establishes budget (may have line item veto on decisions of first-line administrator); negotiates contracts with third party payers and others	Allocates full-time equivalent employees among departments; ensures compliance with employment laws	Approves purchase of equipment and supplies; selects architect, contractors, and so on for building projects; ensures compliance with regulatory certifications	Analyzes data from many sources to prepare reports, advise chief executive officer, and ensure compliance with accreditation and licensure regulations
Chief executive officer (e.g., president)	Promotes fund raising; identifies collaborators, partners, and stakeholders (those who can affect or are affected by the achievement of an organization's objectives) for the organization; answers to board of directors, investors, and shareholders	Hires vice presidents; oversees delegation of responsibilities	Has little, if any, responsibility for operations	Analyzes and shares information with stakeholders and/or shareholders; conducts strategic planning and sets long-range goals based on information provided

Table 8-3 | **Control Exercised at Different Management Levels in Physical Therapy**

Management Level	Control of Own Actions	Control of Others' Future Actions	Direct Control over Work of Others	Control of Goals of Organization	Interaction with Others at Same Level
Patient/client management (i.e., staff physical therapist)	High	Low	High	Indirect; actions lead to goal accomplishment; low level of control in establishment of goals	Varies; may have no contact with other physical therapists (PTs), or extensive interaction may be required to manage caseload
First-line manager (e.g., supervisor, administrator)	High	Moderate	Moderate	Moderate	Minimal
Mid-level manager (e.g., director, vice president)	Very high	High	Low	High	Moderate
Chief executive officer (e.g., president)	Very high	Very high	Minimal	Very high	N/A

N/A, *Not applicable.*

Billing for Physical Therapy Services

The primary financial responsibilities at the patient/client management level of administration is billing for physical therapy services provided. All medical billing is based on the *Current Procedural Terminology* (CPT), which is published by the American Medical Association (AMA).[5] The CPT, first published in 1966, is a list of descriptive terms and identifying codes used to report medical services and procedures. Because it provides a uniform language for describing all medical, surgical, and diagnostic services, the CPT serves as a nationwide means of communication among physicians, patients, and third-party payers. In the 1980s the Health Care Financing Administration (currently the Center for Medicare and Medicaid Services) adopted the CPT for Medicare and Medicaid programs, and it is the preferred coding system of other insurers.[5]

The CPT is not a static text. For example, the fourth edition, published in 1977, included significant updates in medical technology, and periodic updating was initiated to keep pace with the rapidly changing medical environment. This updating continues today.[5] An AMA editorial panel is responsible for revising, updating, and modifying the CPT. The panel, which is composed of 16 multidisciplinary members and an insurance representative, includes a PT, who represents the nonmedical professions.

Just because a service has a CPT code does not mean the PT will be reimbursed for it. Insurors' payment policies determine the language of benefits packages, which are driven by cost containment. PTs, therefore, must remain up-to-date on third-party payer decisions on covered services so that therapists can correlate billing codes accurately with the services provided in each treatment session and also so that they know which services are billable to which insurance companies. Recent issues related to CPT coding for PTs include the following:

- Definition of one-on-one and group therapy
- Use of codes for evaluation and reevaluation
- Billing for interventions and evaluations on the same day
- Denial of reimbursement for physical agents which have been determined to be unskilled

Health professionals may use any CPT code that is within their scope of practice. PTs most often use the 97000 category (i.e., physical medicine and rehabilitation) to bill for their services (Box 8-1). Other professionals, such as physicians, occupational therapists, and chiropractors, also may bill for interventions in this category, and PTs may use codes in other applicable categories.

In addition to specific procedures, the 97000 category includes services measured in time spent with the patient (e.g., 97530, therapeutic activities with direct patient contact, each 15 minutes). The number of units billed under the 97530 code depends on how long the PT was in direct contact with the patient engaged in therapeutic activities. However, code 97110—exercises for strength/ endurance/range of motion (ROM)/flexibility—would be billed as 1 unit regardless of how long the patient exercised.

Payers use a variety of methods to determine the value of each CPT code, such as *contracted rates* (a discount rate negotiated by the payer and a provider, such as a managed care organization) or *capitated rates* (a fixed amount per patient accepted periodically by a provider for services to patients covered by the insurer). More commonly, reimbursement rates are determined by fee schedules. The most frequently used fee schedule is the Resource-Based Relative Value Scale (RBRVS), which is

Box **8-1** CPT Codes Commonly Used by Physical Therapists

Procedures Requiring Constant Attendance

97034 Application modality to 1 area; contrast baths, each 15 min
97032 Electrical stimulation (manual), each 15 min
97036 Hubbard tank, each 15 min
97033 Iontophoresis, each 15 min
97035 Ultrasound, each 15 min
97039 Unlisted modality

Evaluation Procedures

97005 Athletic training evaluation
97006 Athletic training reevaluation
97003 Occupational therapy evaluation
97004 Occupational therapy reevaluation
97001 Physical therapy evaluation
97002 Physical therapy reevaluation

Procedures That Are Supervised Modalities

97010 Application modality more than 1; hot/cold packs
97024 Diathermy
97014 Electrical stimulation
97026 Infrared
97020 Microwave
97018 Paraffin bath
97012 Traction (mechanical)
97028 Ultraviolet
97016 Vasopneumatic devices
97022 Whirlpool

Tests and Measurements

97703 Check out orthotic/prosthetic use, established patient, each 15 min
95875 Ischemic limb exercise test
97750 Physical performance test/measurements with report, each 15 min

Therapeutic Procedures

97537 Community/work reintegration training, 1-on-l, each 15 min
97532 Development cognitive skill, direct patient contact, each 15 min
97140 Manual therapy technique, more than 1 region, each 15 min
97504 Orthotic fitting and training, upper and lower extremities and/or trunk, each 15 min
97520 Prosthesis training, upper and lower extremities, each 15 min
97535 Self-care/home management training, 1-on-1, each 15 min
97533 Sensory integration techniques, direct patient contact, each 15 min
97530 Therapeutic activities, direct patient contact, each 15 min
97113 Therapeutic procedures, more than 1 area, each 15 min; aquatic therapy with therapeutic exercises
97110 Exercises for strength/endurance/range of motion/flexibility
97116 Gait training
97124 Massage, including effleurage, petrissage, and/or tapotement
97112 Neuromuscular reeducation of movement/balance/coordination/kinesthetic sense/posture/proprioception
97150 Therapeutic procedure group
97542 Wheelchair management/propel training, each 15 min
97545 Work hardening/conditioning; initial 2 hr
97546 Each additional hour

Box **8-1**   Cᴘᴛ Cᴏᴅᴇꜱ Cᴏᴍᴍᴏɴʟʏ Uꜱᴇᴅ ʙʏ Pʜʏꜱɪᴄᴀʟ Tʜᴇʀᴀᴘɪꜱᴛꜱ—ᴄᴏɴᴛ'ᴅ

Wound Care Management

97602 Removal of devitalized tissue from wound; nonselective debridement without anesthesia with scissors, scalpel, and tweezers, including topical applications, assessment, and instruction per session

97601 Selective debridement without anesthesia, wet-to-moist dressing, enzyme, abrasion, including topicals, applications, assessment, and instruction per session

---

Modified from *CPT Fast Finder 2003*. Eden Prairie, Minn: Ingenix, Inc.; 2002. Prepared with copyright permission from the American Medical Association.
CPT, Current Procedural Terminology.

used by Medicare. In this system the value of a procedure identified by a CPT code is determined by the following:

- The value of the provider's work, evaluated on the basis of time, technical skill, physical effort, mental effort, and judgment, as well as the psychological stress that may result when the work has a high risk to cause harm to the patient
- Practice expense related to performance of the procedure
- Malpractice costs
- A geographic price cost index (GPCI), which is applied to each of the preceding components to account for economic variations across the United States
- An annual conversion factor, which is used to calculate the amount the provider will be paid for each procedure and is determined annually by Congress and the Centers for Medicare and Medicaid Services (CMS).[6]

Other payers may use the RBRVS to establish a fee schedule, but they often establish conversion factors different from those Medicare uses.

Documentation

The APTA's *Interactive Guide to Physical Therapist Practice with Catalog of Tests and Measures*[1] (commonly known simply as the Guide), defines *documentation* as "any entry into the patient/client record, such as consultation reports, initial examination reports, progress notes, flowsheets, checklists, reexamination reports, or summations of care, that identifies the care or services provided."[1] PTs are responsible for all documentation of the services provided to each patient, even when support personnel actually make the entries and provide the care. This responsibility includes reconciling documentation entries with fees claimed for services provided.

Reimbursement for physical therapy may be *prospective;* that is, the number of sessions and interventions are agreed on prior to initiation of services. In such cases, documentation to justify physical therapy charges may be less important; however, a PT who might want authorization to continue services would be wise to keep records that reflect the three traditional demands of Medicare; specifically, the documentation should show that the services provided were skilled, medically necessary, and related to improvement of function (Table 8-4).

Correct	Incorrect
Patient is unable to follow one-step commands consistently during gait training. Patient's responses to simple questions are inconsistent or not relevant to the questions asked.	Patient is confused and not a good rehabilitation candidate.
Patient initiates appropriate conversation and questions. Recall of instructions from previous treatment session now requires only minimal cueing during functional training.	Patient appears to be getting better.
Patient was asked to demonstrate home exercises. Patient stated she lost the instruction sheet and has not performed exercises as instructed at last visit. Patient was advised of importance of carryover and reinstructed in home program.	Patient is noncompliant.
Odor of alcohol detected on patient's breath, speech slurred, gait unsteady (patient fell against wall in hallway); patient attempted to hug and kiss PT. PT advised patient that his behavior is inappropriate for professional/patient relationship and is interfering with accomplishment of established goals because he is unable to participate in treatment sessions (falls asleep during exercise). Patient advised that another PT, Mr. Smith, has agreed to continue his treatment effective 5/12/04, with Dr. Jones's approval. Patient apologized, stated that he needed help with his drinking, and promised to see Mr. Smith. Patient was given the telephone number of the local Alcoholics Anonymous group and instructed to call Dr. Jones for a referral for counseling.	Patient appears drunk and is disruptive during therapy and makes therapist uncomfortable. D/C.
External rotation of right shoulder continues to be 25/45 degrees with patient expression of 8/10 pain when passive range is attempted. However, patient was observed adjusting a hair clip, which required range of more than 25/45.	Patient is obviously malingering and not trying to move the shoulder to maximum possible range.
Patient takes initiative and reports performing exercise two times since last session. ROM of left knee is −15 to 80 degrees. Patient is able to walk with walker PWB on left leg for 60 feet with occasional verbal cues for heel strike and knee extension.	Patient is pleasant and cooperative and enjoys the treatments. She continues to improve.
Patient performed 30 repetitions each of active exercise of right shoulder in all planes with no complaints of pain during exercise. She reported she was able to drive to the treatment session with her husband as passenger to ensure safety.	Patient received treatment. Tolerated well. Voices no complaints.
1/1/04 9:15 AM Left message for Dr. Neerdowell concerning Mr. Hall's dizziness. 1/1/04 4:45 PM Dr. Neerdowell stated he would write an order to decrease dosage of diovan. 1/2/04 10:30 AM Patient continues to complain of dizziness. Reports that Dr. Neerdowell has not notified her of change in her medication.	Called Dr. Neerdowell for the fourth time; he still has not responded to concerns expressed about Mr. Hall's dizziness, which leaves patient unable to participate in program.

Table 8-4   **Examples of Correct and Incorrect Physical Therapy Documentation***—cont'd

Correct	Incorrect
3/15/04 1 PM Patient was discharged to home on 3/13/04. Goals of safe, supervision only, NWB gait with walker for 50 feet, set for completion on 3/31/04, were not met. PT had no opportunity to instruct caregiver in safe management of wheelchair, transfers, and gait.	D/C note: Patient discharged by UR nurse over the weekend against advice of this PT. Patient is unsafe and too sick to be at home.
5/1/04 10:30 AM Contacted by Mrs. Lewis, daughter of patient; she is concerned about her mother's report that physical therapy sessions are too fatiguing. Explained to Mrs. Lewis that her mother is participating in short bouts of exercise with extended rest between bouts to accommodate for her decreased endurance. Reported to her that her mother is on target with her physical therapy goals and needs encouragement to participate.	Discussed patient with her daughter.
6/15/04 4:30 PM Call to patient, who reported he forgot his appointment this morning. Reminded him to follow exercise program as instructed and rescheduled for 3/16/04.	No show, rescheduled.
9/8/04 11:00 AM Instructed patient and wife in standard TKR postoperative program on file. Patient and wife were able to demonstrate all exercises, transfers, and application of heat as needed.	HEP instruction.
11/21/04 3:30 PM Received verbal order from Dr. Wilson to initiate weight bearing as tolerated on LLE. Initiated orders in parallel bars. Patient unable to achieve heel-toe foot placement and is fearful of accepting weight on LLE.	VO for WBAT.

ROM, *Range of motion;* PWB, *partial weight bearing;* UR, *utilization review;* NWB, *non-weight-bearing;* TKA, *total knee arthroplasty;* HEP, *home exercise program;* LLE, *left lower extremity.*

**Correct physical therapy documentation is specific, objective, related to function, and consistent with general rules. Do not use jargon (e.g., BTB [back to bed] or VO for WBAT [verbal order for weight bearing as tolerated]), and do not use acronyms with more than one meaning (e.g., D/C may mean discharged or discontinued).*

The PT must provide documentation that accurately describes the care provided and supports the need for such care. The following are questions PTs must ask themselves in developing their plans of care:

- Are the treatments specific and effective for the problems identified and the functional goals established?
- Is the patient's condition such that only PTs or personnel they supervise could provide the care?
- Can the patient be expected to reach the established goals within a reasonable time?
- Is the plan of care timely in terms of frequency and duration of service?

The medical record (i.e., documentation) not only supports the charges for services provided, but it also is a legal document. Should harm come to a patient who claims malpractice, the medical record becomes the defense of the health care providers. In addition, both internal monitoring committees and outside institutional accrediting bodies use the medical record retrospectively to analyze the

Box 8-2   **GENERAL RULES OF DOCUMENTATION**

Timeliness

- Try to complete documentation during the intervention session or soon after; it saves time and ensures accuracy.

Objectivity

- Do not record opinions, conclusions, or personal feelings or make judgments about patients. Also, do not use vague words that can mean different things to different people (e.g., better, worse, withdrawn, confused, appears to, apparently, seems).
- Use words that describe the patient's actions. Record only what you see, hear, feel, or smell, what you do for the patient, and how the patient responds. State only the facts, and quote the patient. Do not draw conclusions.

Legibility

- Illegible writing reduces credibility and arouses suspicion; it implies careless, rushed efforts. Unclear writing is a reflection of unclear thinking.

Thoroughness

- Do not leave any blank spaces in the record; if you do not complete a page, draw a large line through the unused space. Be sure to complete any blocks provided to reduce the risk of an addition being made later that could change the information. Use checklists, grids, and flowsheets with caution.
- Mark with your initials rather than check marks to reduce the risk that entries made by others will be taken as yours.
- Document all telephone calls, instructions given to patients, discussions with families, and verbal orders from physicians (signed within 24 hours). If a patient misses an appointment, note it in writing and follow up. Document the reason. Make sure you have a policy regarding cancellations, because large gaps in treatment may jeopardize reimbursement.

Accuracy

- Make sure that all documentation matches billing, attendance grids, and other reports. Inaccurate transferal of dates and numbers reduces credibility and could result in reimbursement and legal problems.
- Use correct spelling and grammar.
- Use abbreviations that are consistent within a work setting and that have a single meaning. Avoid jargon that other PTs, health care providers, or lay individuals will not understand.
- Do not skip lines or white out, erase, or obliterate text. If you make a mistake, draw one line through it and write the word "error" with your initials, *or* write a separate entry as an addendum to a note or a correction.

Meaningfulness

- Do not write for the sake of writing something. If an item doesn't mean anything or doesn't contribute to the information about the patient, don't waste time writing it down. Always consider justification of continued stay in progress notes and leave room to note a change in your thinking or unexpected circumstances.

Professional Courtesy

- Do not use the medical record for complaints, criticism, or arguments with other health care team members.

Box **8-2**   **GENERAL RULES OF DOCUMENTATION—CONT'D**

Authenticity

- *Write your own notes; do not sign someone else's notes.* Co-signing notes arouses suspicion; only the person who provides the service can write the note. (However, co-signing is a commonly accepted practice for instructors supervising students.) Each entry in the record must have a date, time, and legal signature. Many advocate also recording the time the care was provided. Include your license number and professional designation.
- If you continue an entry to another page, your signature must appear at the bottom of the first entry with the word *Continue.* Each page of a multipage form must be signed and dated.
- Other rules in organizational policies and procedures apply for authentication of electronic documentation.

Decision-Making Process

- Make sure the documentation reflects the ways patient progress and interventions are linked to examination data and evaluation.
- Document the patient's response to treatment, as well as modifications of care based on that response.
- Make sure the documentation reflects the continuity of care among providers and communication among all caregivers.
- Make sure the reason for discharge is clear.

---

quality of care. The principles of documentation (Box 8-2) apply, regardless of the practice setting or documentation system.

Many health care systems have incorporated centralized information systems, which allow providers to make their documentation entries through a computer. The entries are transmitted to the medical record, which can be accessed by all providers involved with the patient's care. These systems have alleviated some of the problems associated with the traditional manual-entry method. Computer-based documentation has the potential to do the following:

- Reduce the time spent on documentation and thereby maximize the provision of direct patient care
- Eliminate duplication and reduce entry errors
- Limit entries to specific required information
- Improve the timeliness of the information shared
- Provide prompts for required entries

However, computer-based documentation also presents new challenges in terms of patient privacy, confidentiality of information, and security of records. The APTA has established guidelines for documentation and recommended documentation forms that are consistent with the terminology, patient/client management model, and practice patterns of the Guide.[1]

Persuading all PTs to use the same documentation forms is a challenge because use of the APTA forms is voluntary and requires some familiarity with the Guide. Also, the documentation submitted for Medicare billing is not consistent with the APTA's recommended terminology, and PTs are not likely to adopt two formats that would result in duplication of effort.

Despite these obstacles, standard terminology and documentation formats are important for communication, not only between PTs themselves but also among PTs and other health care providers, third-party payers, attorneys, and accrediting agencies. From a research standpoint, standardized terminology and documentation formats would be a major advantage in building a knowledge base from clinical data.

Direction and Supervision of Support Personnel

According to the *Guide,* "Direction and supervision are essential to the provision of high-quality physical therapy."[1] Several factors determine which tasks should be delegated and the extent to which support personnel must be supervised:

- The education and experience of the person supervised
- The type of organization in which the work is performed
- The applicable state law
- The task to be performed

The APTA has identified three levels of supervision that the PT may provide[7]:

- *General supervision:* The PT is not required to be on site for direction and supervision but at the least must be available by some form of telecommunication like phone or pager.
- *Direct supervision:* The PT is physically present and immediately available for direction and supervision. The PT has direct contact with the patient during each visit (defined in the *Guide* as all encounters with a patient in a 24-hour period).[1] Availability by telecommunication does not meet the requirement of direct supervision.
- *Direct personal supervision:* The PT or, when allowed by law, the PTA is physically present and immediately available to direct and supervise tasks related to patient/client management. Direction and supervision are continuous throughout the performance of the tasks. Availability by telecommunication does not meet the requirement of direct personal supervision.

The most important guides for decisions on delegation and supervision are the state practice acts, which define and set rules for physical therapy practice in each state. Practice acts vary widely (Box 8-3), and Medicare has its own regulations on supervision (Table 8-5).

Ultimately, as the Florida practice act states, "The delegation of tasks and direction of actions to subordinates is a serious responsibility for the physical therapist. The primary concern of the physical therapist is always the safety, well-being, and best interest of the patient."[8] PTs use their professional expertise to determine which components of the plan of care can be delegated because the PT is also responsible for maximizing the availability of physical therapy services. This is accomplished by direct delivery of services by PTs with responsible use of PTAs, who assist with specific components of care.

Another category of physical therapy personnel are the physical therapy aides. Aides are any support personnel who perform designated tasks related to the operation of the physical therapy service; if those tasks are related to patient/client management and are allowed by law, they must be performed only under the direct personal supervision of the PT or PTA (i.e., the PT or PTA must be physically present and immediately available to continuously direct and supervise the tasks). In such cases the PT or PTA is expected to have direct contact with the patient during each session. An aide most appropriately may be considered an extra pair of hands during a treatment session, rather than an individual to whom any part of the plan of care could be delegated.

In most jurisdictions anyone who is not licensed under the physical therapy practice act is considered an aide (aides may also be called *technicians*), although the aide may be licensed under other practice acts. For example, athletic trainers and massage therapists, although they may be licensed in their disciplines, are not licensed under physical therapy practice acts. As a general rule, legally and in terms of

Box 8-3   SUPERVISION AND DELEGATION IN FIVE STATES

New York

- PTA works under the supervision of a licensed physical therapist (PT), performing such patient-related activities as are assigned by the supervising PT. Supervision of a PTA by a licensed physical therapist shall be on-site supervision but not necessarily direct personal supervision.
- Information Web site: www.op.nysed.gov/article136.htm

Washington

- The PT is professionally and legally responsible for patient care given by supportive personnel under the PT's supervision. If a PT fails to adequately supervise patient care given by supportive personnel, disciplinary action may be taken against the physical therapist.
- The number of full-time equivalent PTAs and aides used in any physical therapy practice shall not exceed twice the number of full-time equivalent licensed PTs practicing therein.
- The PTA may function under direct or indirect supervision. Reevaluation must be performed by a supervising licensed PT every five visits; or reevaluation must be performed at least once a week if treatment is received more than five times a week; or reevaluation is required when there is any change in the patient's condition not consistent with planned progress or treatment goals.
- Information Web site: www.leg.wa.gov/wac/index.cfm?fuseaction=chapterdigest&chapter=246-915

Illinois

- The PTA works under general supervision of a licensed PT to assist in implementing the physical therapy treatment. The PT must maintain continual contact with the PTA, including periodic personal supervision and instruction to ensure the safety and welfare of the patient. The term "physical therapy aide" means a person who has received on-the-job training specific to the facility. Aides must perform patient care activities under the on-site supervision of a license PT or licensed PTA. Disciplinary action is taken when PTAs interpret referrals; perform evaluation, procedures, or planning; or make major modifications of patient programs; or when a PTA or supervising PT fails to maintain continued contact.
- Information Web site: www.legis.state.il.us/legislation/ilcs/ch225/ch225act90.htm

Arizona

- Assistive personnel include PTAs, physical therapy aides, and other trained or educated health care providers who perform designated tasks under the direct supervision of a PT.
- A PT shall determine and document the assistive personnel's education and training before delegating.
- For each date of service, a PT shall provide all therapeutic interventions that require the expertise of a PT and shall determine whether the use of assistive personnel to deliver services is safe, effective, and efficient for each patient.
- A PT shall concurrently supervise no more than three assistive personnel. If three assistive personnel are supervised, at least one shall be a PTA.
- Information Web site: www.ptboard.state.az.us/

Georgia

- Licensed PTs shall at all times be responsible for providing adequate supervision of assistants supervised by them. The licensed PT shall be present in the same institutional setting 50% of any workweek or the portion thereof the assistant is on duty and shall be readily available to the assistant at all other times for advice, assistance, and instruction. In the home health setting, the PT responsible for the patient shall supervise the PTA working

Continued

Box 8-3   **Supervision and Delegation in Five States—Cont'd**

with the patient and shall meet with the assistant no less than once weekly to review all patients being treated, document all meetings with the assistant and subsequent decisions, make an on-site visit to each patient treated by the assistant as appropriate, based on the need to alter the treatment plan, at least every sixth visit. In the school setting, a PT must be designated as the PTA's supervisor and must make an on-site visit to each student scheduled for direct weekly services from the PTA no less than every fourth scheduled week, and no less than once every 3 months for students who are scheduled with the PTA once monthly or less and be available to the PTA at all times for advice, assistance, and instructions.
- Adequate supervision by a licensed PT shall include interaction with the assistant in appropriate ways specific to the plan of care of the patients being treated by the assistant.
- Information Web site: www.ganet.org/rules/index.cgi?base=490/5/01

provision of skilled physical therapy services, they are not practicing physical therapy and their services cannot be billed as physical therapy, although they may be working in a physical therapy service.

Some third-party payers have argued that delegation of an intervention to support personnel implies that the procedure does not require the skilled services of a PT, and reimbursement has been denied for services provided by any support personnel, including PTAs. This raises the concern that if PTs must do all the work of patient care, they may be assuming more technical tasks than their skills and training require and, as a result, patient goals will not be accomplished in the most cost-effective manner. PTs must therefore be very careful to clarify that the PTA's work is an extension of the skilled service of the PT. PTs also must be well versed in the state statutes that govern their practice and in Medicare and other third-party interpretations of skilled physical therapy services.

First-Line Management

First-line managers in physical therapy may be assigned direct patient care tasks in addition to financial, operations, human resource, and information responsibilities. Their duties include budgeting; hiring, firing, and evaluating staff members; and ensuring that the organization meets accreditation, certification, and other legal requirements.

Budget Responsibilities

Budgeting is the process of making decisions about revenue and expenses to ensure that funds are available to meet the goals of the organization. A first-line manager may be asked to contribute to this decision-making process, which may occur annually, biannually, or even at 5-year intervals. More important, first-line managers are held accountable for implementing the components of an organization's budget that apply to physical therapy services. A first-line manager may report on revenue and expenses to a midlevel manager as often as weekly. More typically, budget projections are formally reviewed monthly with the midlevel manager, who may oversee coordination of the budget among several departments.

Table 8-5 | **Medicare Supervision Requirements for Physical Therapist Assistants**

Facility or Agency	*Requirements*
Certified rehabilitation agency (CRA)	Qualified personnel must provide the initial direction for, as well as periodic observation of, the actual performance of the function or activity. If the person providing services does not meet the qualifications of an assistant-level practitioner, the physical therapist (PT) must be on the premises.
Comprehensive outpatient rehabilitation facility (CORF)	Services must be provided by qualified personnel. If personnel do not meet Medicare qualifications, qualified staff members must be on the premises and must instruct the providers in appropriate patient care service and techniques; the qualified staff members are responsible for the service providers' activities. A qualified professional must be on the premises of the facility or must be available through direct telecommunication for consultation and assistance during the facility's operating hours.
Home health agencies (HHA)	Services must be performed safely and effectively and only by or under the general supervision of a skilled PT. Health Care Financing Administration manuals traditionally have defined "general supervision" as requiring initial direction and periodic inspection of the actual activity. However, the supervisor need not always be physically present or on the premises when the physical therapist assistant (PTA) is providing services.
Inpatient and outpatient hospital services	Services must be performed safely and effectively and only by or under the supervision of a qualified PT. Because the regulations do not specify the types of direction required, the provider must defer to the individual state's physical therapy practice act.
Physical therapist in private practice (PTPP)	Services must be provided by or under the personal supervision of the PT in private practice. In the PTPP setting, the physical therapist must be in the room when the PTA provides a service.
Physician's office	Services must be provided under the physician's direct supervision. The physician must be in the office suite when an individual procedure is performed by support personnel.
Skilled nursing facility (SNF)	Skilled rehabilitation services must be provided directly by or under the general supervision of skilled rehabilitation personnel. "General supervision" requires initial direction and periodic inspection of the actual activity. However, the supervisor need not always be physically present or on the premises when the PTA performs the service.

First-line managers are responsible for ensuring that projected revenue is met and that projected expenses are not exceeded. The major source of revenue, reimbursement for services provided, is analyzed in terms of the projected *payer mix* (i.e., which payer accounts for what percentage of revenue) and the fee schedules for each payer or contract (Figure 8-3). The typical categories of expenses are salaries and benefits, Federal Insurance Contributions Act (Social Security) payments, recruitment, equipment, and supplies. A freestanding facility or practice also has budget provisions for professional services, rent or lease, utilities, telephone service, maintenance, depreciation, and insurance. In large organizations some of these expenses may be prorated to departments on the basis of square footage, the number of employees, or some other formula by which expenses are shared across the board.

Revenue

Gross Revenue: _____

   Services*: _____

   Equipment: _____

Less Deductions: _____

Non-Operating Revenue: _____

Total Revenue: _____

Expenses

Salaries: _____

Benefits: _____

FICA: _____

Education: _____

Recruitment: _____

Professional Services: _____

Purchased Services: _____

Supplies: _____

Travel: _____

Dues: _____

Equipment: _____

Rent/Lease: _____

Utilities: _____

Communication: _____

Environmental Services: _____

Insurance: _____

Total Expenses: _____

Net Income
(Total Revenue – Total Expenses): _____

Taxes: _____

Net Income After Taxes: _____

*Payer Mix: Medicare (28%), Medicaid (1%), Managed Care (29%), Commercial (22%), Charity (1%), Self Pay (19%)

Figure 8-3. Sample budget with payer mix (i.e., the percentage of the budget accounted for by each payer). (*From Nosse LJ, Friberg DG, Kovacek PR. Managerial and supervisory principles for physical therapists. Baltimore: Williams & Wilkins; 1999.*)

Operations Responsibilities

First-level managers are responsible for capital equipment decisions. Allocation of these funds is part of the budgeting process, although it is considered separately. Typically, equipment is considered a capital investment at some predetermined cost (e.g., over $1000). Because funds for capital investment frequently are limited, managers often must submit a cost/benefit analysis to determine the potential gain in meeting the organization's goals (see Case Scenario 4).

Other operations responsibilities may include assigning staff members to particular units or patients, determining the ratio of PTs to support staff (i.e., the skill mix), and establishing productivity goals (Table 8-6). These decisions are closely tied to budget determinations because salaries and benefits are always the greatest expenses. First-line managers are responsible for striking a balance between use of the least expensive (and least skilled) individuals able to provide care and maintenance of the quality of care.

Human Resource Responsibilities

The human resource responsibilities of first-line managers include the hiring, firing, and evaluation of staff members, decisions that are affected by a number of federal employment laws. In large organizations human resource experts assist in the management of many of these employment factors. However, the first-line manager may have some control over salary negotiations and a great deal of responsibility for assignment and scheduling of staff members, payroll reporting, and evaluation of performance, which usually is linked to salary increases. Fairness and consistency in these matters are not only legally important, but they are also vital to staff morale.

Information Responsibilities

A major responsibility of the first-line manager is training staff members in correct documentation and supervising all record keeping. Often this task is integrated into

Table 8-6 | **Survey of Productivity Expectations for Physical Therapists**[*]

	STANDARD		
Type of Practice *Patient Care*	*Hours of Direct* *Patient Care*	*Number of* *Patients Seen*	*Number of Visits* *Completed*
Acute care	21.0[†]	27.5	33.7
Subacute care	26.0	21.6	40.5
Health care patient	26.5	34.7	40.5
Private outpatient	34.2	42.7	51.7
Skilled nursing facility, extended care and intermediate care facilities	43.4	25.9	34.2
Home care	20.9	15.8	23.6

Adapted from American Physical Therapy Association. Mean productivity expectations by practice setting. Retrieved December 1, 2004, at http://www.apta.org/Documents/Membersonly/Research/ProductivityExpertPT.pdf. This material is copyrighted, and any further reproduction or distribution is prohibited.

[*]*Respondents were full-time employees, and the data reflect 1 week of work.*

[†]*Mean (n).*

other quality assurance processes. As part of the Health Insurance Portability and Accountability Act (HIPAA), recent federal legislation has tightened the rules protecting the confidentiality and security of patient information (Box 8-4).

Another major information responsibility of the first-line manager is preparation of regular reports (typically quarterly) to mid-level managers that provide information on issues such as productivity, budget status, ongoing projects, and progress toward meeting departmental goals. Depending on the type of organization, first-line managers are also responsible for contributing to the preparation of materials required for accreditation and licensure of organizations and compliance with the numerous health care regulations. The APTA standards of practice are an important source of information on these issues for first-line physical therapy managers.[19]

First-line managers face many challenges. Their jobs are difficult because they answer to a number of work initiators who are higher or lower in rank. Guy[10] described this difficulty as the conflict-ridden position of the person in the middle. At this management level, more discord is seen among managers themselves,

---

Box 8-4   HEALTH INSURANCE PORTABILITY AND ACCOUNTABILITY ACT

The Health Insurance Portability and Accountability Act (HIPAA) of 1996 has two components:
1. The *administrative simplification rule,* which requires standardization of forms and allows full electronic transactions for Medicare claims, including forms for health claims or encounter information, health claim attachments, enrollment and disenrollment, eligibility for a health plan, payment and remittance advice, health plan premium payments, first report of injury, health claim status, referral certification, and authorization.
2. The *privacy rule,* which provides comprehensive federal protection for the privacy of health information. The rule does not replace federal, state, or other laws that afford even greater privacy protections and does not interfere with patient access to or the quality of health care services. Provisions of the privacy rule include the following:
   - The average health care plan or health care provider must (1) notify patients of their privacy rights and the ways their information can be used; (2) adopt and implement privacy procedures; (3) designate an individual to be responsible for ensuring that privacy procedures are adopted and followed; (4) make sure employees are trained in privacy procedures; and (5) secure patient records containing individually identifiable health information.
   - Covered entities must make reasonable efforts to limit the use or disclosure of and requests for protected health information to the minimum necessary to accomplish the intended purpose.
   - Covered entities must implement appropriate administrative, technical, and physical safeguards to reasonably preserve protected health information (PHI) from any intentional or unintentional use or disclosure that violates the privacy rule. PHI includes individually identifiable health information in any form, including information transmitted orally or in written or electronic form. Examples of reasonable safeguards include (1) speaking quietly when discussing a patient's condition in the waiting room with the family; (2) avoiding the use of patients' names in public hallways; (3) locking file cabinets or records rooms; and (4) providing additional passwords on computers.
   - Covered entities may use and disclose PHI without the patient's consent for treatment, payment, and health care operations activities.

Modified from American Physical Therapy Association. *Privacy regulations.* Retrieved November 9, 2003, at http://www.apta.org/Govt_Affairs/regulatory/fraud_abuse/hipaa/Privacy. *This material is copyrighted, and any further reproduction or distribution is prohibited.*

regardless of the mix of disciplines, and managers agree less with each other than at lower or higher management levels.[10]

Guy[10] also found that professional credentials elevate an individual in an organization and evoke a sense that the person's beliefs and values are valid. However, once the individual has achieved a managerial position, rank rather than professional status influences the perception of the person's values and decisions. The more complex an organization, the wider the spectrum of any set of considerations, the more varied the staff members' views, and the more numerous the alternatives to be considered. Also, the variety of pressures and influences on staff members increases. Thus, as complexity increases, so does the baseline of conflict across professions. More factors must be considered and more preferences accommodated.

Midlevel Managers and Chief Executive Officers

The responsibilities of the midlevel manager and chief executive officer have little to do with day-to-day patient care and management of services; at these higher levels of management, decisions must be made about the organization as a whole and its interaction with other organizations. Individuals at this level of management are concerned with the following:

- Negotiating contracts with third-party payers and subcontractors
- Establishing goals for the organization
- Identifying partners, collaborators, and stakeholders who affect those goals
- Ensuring the organization's compliance with accreditation, licensure, and other regulations
- Communicating with boards of trustees and shareholders
- Marketing the organization
- Safeguarding the organization's financial solvency

PTs who hold these higher level management positions often have graduate degrees in health care or business administration or have been trained through corporate staff development programs. They may find themselves far removed from the practice of physical therapy. The exception is the PT who establishes a private practice and thereby assumes responsibility for all levels of management, including patient/client management. Exciting, independent practice opportunities abound for entrepreneurial PTs who have strong patient care and managerial skills.

Leadership

As can be seen in Table 8-1, leadership theories have evolved because of the wide range of perspectives from which leaders can be viewed. Leaders have not really changed; groups of people still need leadership, and every group has a leader. Our understanding of leadership depends on the perspective, be it the characteristics of leaders, the roles of leaders, or the process of becoming a leader.

An underlying premise is that the organizational structure, management style, and leadership style all must mesh if an organization is to meet its goals efficiently and effectively. For example, a great man (or great woman) leadership style in an organization supported by work teams in a participative management model would result in confusion about who is in charge, how decisions are made, and who is accountable for the outcomes of the organization's work. Transitions from one organizational model to another are made with great difficulty and are determined by the organization's leadership. Strong leadership also explains why traditional organizations remain successful; leaders can motivate and control to achieve goals.

ETHICAL AND LEGAL ISSUES

APTA Code of Ethics and Guide for Professional Conduct

The APTA's *Code of Ethics* rarely refers to the administrative role of the physical therapist. For example, Principle 6 of the code states that "[a] physical therapist shall maintain and promote high standards for physical therapy practice, education, and research" but does not refer to the administrative or consultant roles.[10] The principles of the code that most directly relate to the role of the administrator are 3 (compliance with laws and regulations), 4 (exercise of sound judgment), 7 (reasonable and deserved remuneration), 8 (accurate and relevant information), and 9 (protecting the public). Principle 3 states, "A physical therapist shall comply with laws and regulations governing physical therapy and shall strive to effect changes that benefit patients/clients."[11]

In the APTA's *Guide for Professional Conduct* (GPC), Section 4.2 explicitly addresses direction and supervision, stating that the supervising PT "has primary responsibility for the physical therapy services rendered" (GPC 4.2A).[11] This section also prohibits a PT from delegating "to a less qualified person any activity that requires the professional skill, knowledge, and judgment of the physical therapist" (GPC 4.2B).[12]

The GPC elaborates on Principle 7 of the *Code of Ethics* regarding business arrangements, making it quite clear that PTs must concern themselves with the ethical stance of the organization: "A physical therapist's business/employment practices shall be consistent with the ethical principles of the association" (GPC 7.1A) and "a physical therapist shall never place his/her own financial interest above the welfare of individuals under his/her care"[12] (GPC 7.1B). The GPC lists unacceptable business practices as underutilizing services (GPC 7.1C), overutilizing services (GPC 7.1D), participating in unearned fees (GPC 7.1F), and receiving unearned commission or gratuities (GPC 7.1G). The GPC also states that PTs may ethically participate in the pooling of fees and money (GPC 7.1H), may enter into organizational agreements (GPC 7.1I), may endorse products (GPC 7.2 A-C), and accept payment for endorsements (GPC 7.2 B).[12]

Organizational Ethics

A particularly difficult ethical situation arises for PTs when the ethical standards of their workplace conflict with their professional ethics and values. The GPC states clearly that PTs have an obligation to attempt to resolve conflicts between organizational and professional ethics: "A physical therapist shall advise his/her employer(s) of any employer practice that causes a physical therapist to be in conflict with the ethical principles of the association. A physical therapist shall seek to eliminate aspects of his/her employment that are in conflict with the ethical principles of the association" (GPC 4.3B).[10]

The health care organizations in which PTs work affect physical therapy directly through policies and procedures. Although this direct influence is considerable, organizations may exert even greater influence by creating an organizational culture. Organizational culture refers to the shared beliefs, values, ideas, and expected behaviors within a group entity. As indicated by recent accounting scandals, the organizational culture shapes the ethical decisions and behavior of managers and employees. Because most PTs are salaried employees, they may feel they have no control over business practices or the organizational culture. Some PTs may not even know the fees charged by the organization for their services, and they may be unfamiliar with billing procedures.

A fundamental reason for the frequent conflicts between professional ethics and the ethics of health care institutions is the differing paradigms of medicine and business. The premise of managed care and the current health care system is that health care should be run more efficiently and more cost effectively; that is, more like a business. Although most agree that health care costs must be controlled, business and medicine unquestionably have competing values.

As Mariner[13] points out, business and medicine make different assumptions about relationships with patients, goals, ethical principles, the nature of health care, and the obligations of providers. Business operates on a contractual basis with a "buyer beware" philosophy, and its goal is efficiency and maximization of profit. The guiding ethical principle in business is fair competition in delivering the commodity of health care. In the business model, providers are accountable to stockholders for making the organization profitable.[13]

In contrast, relationships in medicine (and physical therapy) are based on trust rather than contracts. The ethical principles of autonomy (self-determination), beneficence (promoting good), nonmaleficence (preventing harm), and justice guide decision making in medicine, and health is viewed as either a service or a right. In the medical model, the providers' primary obligation is to the patient rather than the organization or stockholders.[13,14] Given the radically different assumptions of the two models, which coexist in the current health care system, conflict between organizational and professional values is not surprising.

The Administrator's Role and Conflict of Interest

Managed care fosters conflict of interest and divided loyalty by creating incentives for cost containment. In addition to the conflicts of interests created by reimbursement incentives, administrators may create conflicts for staff PTs through personnel policies. For example, unrealistic productivity standards or bonuses may force staff PTs to choose between the provision of quality care and their financial self-interests. The first-line manager faces the same challenges for the staff as a whole, which may result in policing rather than leading and developing the staff. Similarly, organizations in financial trouble may adopt policies that are not in the best interest of patients, such as setting limits on the number of visits per patient or directing staff PTs to come up with the most billable units possible for each patient.

More than other employees, first-line managers, caught between the high-level managers making such policies and the staff PTs who provide direct patient care, may feel their loyalty divided between their employers and their professional values. Through their supervision of staff members, first-line managers influence the professional values of many others by example and direction. At the same time, they are responsible on a daily basis for meeting the goals of the organization in terms of productivity, target charges, and other factors. These competing loyalties may be a reason some organizations prefer managers who are not health care professionals.

Whistleblowing

All PTs, whether staff members or managers, may become aware of acts of incompetence, unethical behavior, or illegal activity. Although most people find such actions difficult to report, professionals have an obligation to help regulate colleagues and protect the public. Reporting unethical or illegal behavior is especially difficult when a PT's workplace is involved because employees are expected to be loyal to the organization. In addition, whistleblowers may face negative consequences within the organization. Although a number of state and local laws protect or even encourage whistleblowing, those who report illegal or unethical behavior may be ostracized or denied future opportunities for professional advancement. Coyne[15] recommends the following five steps in approaching this dilemma:

- Self-analysis
- Discussion with the person engaging in unethical behavior
- Approaching a supervisor
- Taking the matter up the managerial ladder
- Filing a complaint

These steps make it clear that other attempts should be made to resolve the issue before the PT resorts to actual whistleblowing.

Perhaps because it is difficult to confront colleagues, licensing boards and ethics committees report that too few PTs report unethical or illegal behavior. This unfortunate reality would seem to be an abdication of the professional responsibility to self-regulate and protect the public.

The Administrator's Role in the Ethics Literature

Only a few peer-reviewed ethics articles published between 1970 and 2000 addressed the PT's role as administrator (see Figure 4-5). Although few publications focused specifically on the ethical issues faced by administrators, several articles that addressed multiple roles included the administrative level.[16]

FURTHER THOUGHTS

Even in staff positions, PTs are managers of their assigned work as they manage resources in the care of patients in relation to their organizations' overall goals. For many of these staff PTs, first-line management promotions are imposed. Others seek these positions. Financial, human resource, operational, and information responsibilities take up much of the time of staff PTs who are responsible for supervising the work of others. Challenges arise from this "person in the middle" position because the first-line manager is responsible for the performance and job satisfaction of staff members, yet is also accountable to higher management for contributing to the organization's goals by implementing the physical therapy program. This often leads to conflicts between professional and business values.

Some PTs assume midlevel manager and chief executive officer positions, typically with additional internal management training or formal graduate studies in business or health care management. Other therapists may take an entrepreneurial approach and develop an independent physical therapy practice, in which they assume all levels of management responsibility.

CASE SCENARIOS

Case Scenario 1

You have an opportunity to explore an alternative organizational structure for the headquarters of the American Physical Therapy Association.
- *Consider the alternatives and justify your choice.*

Case Scenario 2

Charles Yung performed the following treatments during a therapy session with Carla Santini, who had suffered a fracture of the distal humerus and head of the radius of the right arm. Ms. Santini was in physical therapy from 1:05 to 1:45 PM. Charles began the session by reevaluating Carla's right elbow; he discovered that ROM had improved to −10 degrees of extension to 95 degrees of flexion. Supination and pronation remained fixed with the forearm in neutral position. The circumference of the right elbow was 1.5 inches greater than the circumference of the left elbow. Charles noted a trigger point in the extensor complex, and Ms. Santini complained of constant pain that disrupted her sleep. PTA Jim Jackson provided whirlpool and underwater ultrasound treatments to the right elbow and forearm, followed by massage to the upper extremity and passive ROM exercises. Charles reinstructed the patient in self-stretching of the elbow.
- *Complete the following charge slip to reflect this treatment session and then write a note documenting the session.*

Date of Service	CPT CODE	# of Units

- *How many units would be credited to Charles and Jim for productivity for that session?*

Case Scenario 3

The staff of a physical therapy outpatient practice includes two PTs, a PTA, a massage therapist, a certified athletic trainer, and a physical therapy technician.

- *How should the PTs determine the services that could be delegated to the other staff members?*

Case Scenario 4

You need to obtain a .... Complete the form in Box 8-5 to request this piece of equipment.

Case Scenario 5

It is Monday morning, and seven new patients admitted to the hospital over the weekend must be distributed among the four PTs on staff. Everyone on the staff is already working at maximum capacity.

- *As supervisor, how do you decide who gets how many patients and which patients they get?*

Box 8-5   **Equipment Request Form**

General Purpose Capital Equipment Request
Description of item:

_____

_____

Quantity: _____   Unit cost: _____   Total cost: _____
Replacement or new? (If replacement, provide invoice number and date of purchase of item to be replaced.)

_____

_____

_____

Justification
Purpose:

_____

Indicate how purchase affects a critical outcome or mission:

_____

If replacement, explain why current item is no longer usable:

_____

Potential risk if request is not approved:

_____

_____

Case Scenario 6

Two of the four PTs on staff have called in sick with the flu. Dr. Bonnett, one of your best referral sources, has called to say that he is sending over three patients who are in acute pain because of a car accident, and he wants them treated right away.

- *How do you reassign staff members for today?*

Case Scenario 7

You have received a memo from the home office stating your plan for providing physical therapy coverage 365 days per year is due on Monday. You cannot hire more staff members.

- *What plan do you submit?*

Case Scenario 8

One of the PTs you supervise, Selma, is competent, compassionate, and very good with patients. However, despite two warnings about excessive time off (she uses accumulated time off as soon as she has it), she has called in sick again, and she has no time off left.

- *What do you do?*

Case Scenario 9

Robert has been employed as a PT by Riverport Community Hospital for 15 years. For 14 years he believed he had found his "dream" job. A year ago a large health care corporation purchased Riverport and made numerous changes to "improve the bottom line." Robert has been unhappy with this direction, and many other PTs have left for other positions. Over the past few weeks several of Robert's patients have complained about their bills for PT services. Three patients showed him bills with charges that were higher than Robert had submitted or recorded. When he asked the billing officer about this, Robert was told that charges sometimes were adjusted because "the therapists all undercharge." At least one PT has been fired for challenging the new administration's policies.

- *What should Robert do?*

Case Scenario 10

Part of the Health Insurance Portability and Accountability Act of 1996 protects patients' confidential information by limiting access to medical records. You have been charged with ensuring that the physical therapy department is in compliance with this provision.

- *How can you find out the requirements of the law, and how will you ensure compliance?*

REFERENCES

1. American Physical Therapy Association. *The interactive guide to physical therapist practice with catalog of tests and measures* (version 1.0). Alexandria, Va: The Association; 2002.
2. Mark A. Outsourcing therapy services: A strategy for professional autonomy. *Health Manpower Management* 1994;20:37-40.
3. American Physical Therapy Association. *APTA organizational chart.* Retrieved November 9, 2003, at http://www.apta.org/governance/governance_13

4. American Physical Therapy Association. *APTA headquarters organization chart 2002.* Retrieved November 9, 2003, at www.apta.org/governance/governance_13

5. American Medical Association. *The CPT process: How a code becomes a code.* Retrieved November 9, 2003, http://www.ama-assn.org/ama/pub/category/3882.html

6. American Physical Therapy Association. *Medicine reimbursement for physical therapists under resource-based relative value system (RBRVs) during 2002.* Retrieved November 9, 2003, at http://www.apta.org/Govt_Affairs/regulatory/archives/feeschedule/RBRV

7. American Physical Therapy Association. *APTA levels of supervision.* Retrieved November 9, 2003, at http://www.apta.org/PT_Practice/For_Clinicians/Use_of_Personnel_/Levels

8. State of Florida. *Florida statutes: Chapter 64B15.* Retrieved November 9 2003, at http://fac.dos.state.fl.us/faconline/chapter64.pdf

9. American Physical Therapy Association: *Standards of practice.* Available at http://www.apta.org/governance/HOD/policies/HoDpolicies/Section_4/BOD_03041944

10. Guy ME. *Professionals in organizations.* New York: Praeger; 1985.

11. American Physical Therapy Association. *APTA code of ethics.* Retrieved October 27, 2004, at http://www.apta.org/pt_practice/ethics_pt/code_ethics

12. American Physical Therapy Association. *APTA guide for professional conduct.* Retrieved October 27, 2004, at www.apta.org/pt_practice/ethics_pt/pro_conduct

13. Mariner WK. Business versus medical ethics: Conflicting standards for managed care. *J Law Med Ethics* 1995;23:236-246.

14. Swisher LL, Brophy-Krueger C. *Legal and ethical issues in physical therapy.* Woburn, Mass: Butterworth-Heinemann; 1998.

15. Coyne C. Whistleblowing and problem-solving: A 5-step approach. *PT Magazine* 2003;11(2):42-48.

16. Swisher LL. A retrospective analysis of ethics knowledge in physical therapy (1970-2000). *Phys Ther* 2002;82:692-706.

Professionalism in the Multiple Contexts of the U.S. Health Care System

9

[People] are social individuals. Both elements are essential: first, we are unique, irreplaceable individuals; second, our individuality began and can only survive and flourish in social interdependence. We can further make a rough distinction between two levels of social complexity: the larger civic community (nation, state, region) and the smaller, mediating social realities of family, business, and church. This thought model of individuals existing within larger social organizations (family, church, business), which in turn exist within a unifying social entity (state, nation) provides a helpful model for negotiating the hard choices.

—John W. Glaser and Ronald P. Hamel[1]

[N]ew graduates were not expected to have extensive knowledge of or skill in performing the majority of the [management] components included in the categories. We conclude from these results that the respondents expect physical therapists to develop the basis for business-related knowledge and the skill needed for clinical practice after entering clinical practice.

— Rosalie B. Lopopolo, D. Sue Schafer, and Larry J. Nosse[2]

The task of managing a professional complex adaptive system is not to know what is going on and then tell others in the organization what to do. The fundamental unknowability of the system makes this a futile objective. Rather, the task is to create a learning organization. Learning in professional organizations may be remarkably difficult.

— R. A. Anderson and R. R. McDaniel, Jr[3]

THE ORGANIZATIONAL, CULTURAL, SOCIAL, AND POLITICAL CONTEXTS OF HEALTH CARE

The concept of professionalism historically has focused on the relationship between the professional and the individual patient. However, organizational, social, cultural, and political environments clearly have a profound impact on the work of professionals, especially in medicine. Systems and environments shape the ability to fulfill professional roles and the obligations to each patient. In fact, many professional obligations cannot be fulfilled without the establishment of organizational, political, and social policies. Unfortunately, organizations and social systems also have the power to work against social and professional ideals and can contribute to discrimination.

Because organizations and social systems are such integral parts of the health care system, it is important that physical therapists (PTs) understand the ways in which these collective entities may influence their roles. The organizational and cultural contexts of health care give rise to questions such as the following:

1. How do organizations, cultures, and social systems influence the work of the PT?
2. What is meant by the term *cultural competence?* What policies should health care organizations implement to ensure that patient services are culturally appropriate?
3. What is an organizational culture? How does it develop or change? What can PTs do when the organizational culture and their professional obligations conflict?
4. How do individuals, organizations, and systems contribute to discrimination? Why is it important to distinguish between individual prejudice, biased organizational policies, and systemic institutional bias?
5. What can PTs do to shape health care policy? Do they have an obligation to act as advocates for sound policies?
6. What is leadership? Is it different from management? Do professionals have an obligation to be leaders?

This chapter describes the organizational, political, and social environments of the health care system; provides a framework for analyzing health care issues; discusses the importance of a culture for individuals, organizations, and the health care system as a whole; explores different ideas of leadership; distinguishes different levels of discrimination; and suggests strategies for balancing organizational and professional obligations. It also familiarizes the student with organizational terminology (Table 9-1).[4-7]

COMPLEXITY OF THE CURRENT HEALTH CARE SYSTEM

Managed care has made PTs acutely aware that organizations, systems, and environment affect the delivery of health care. When health care services were provided primarily through a fee-for-service system (i.e., professionals were reimbursed for each procedure they performed), the emphasis was on productivity and service to individual patients. However, this model offered few incentives for cost control, and ever-increasing health care costs resulted. The portion of the gross national product (GNP) consumed by health care grew steadily each decade: from 1929 to 1940, the increase was 4%; from 1980 to 1990, it was 12.2%.[8]

Implementation of Medicare and Medicaid legislation in the 1960s resulted in a particularly marked increase in health care spending.[8] Rising concern about the ability of federal and state governments and private companies to subsidize health care produced a growing number of managed care plans, especially after passage of the Health Maintenance Organization Act of 1973.[8]

The numerous strategies used by managed care plans to minimize costs for the system have affected the professional relationship between PTs and their patients.[9] For example, managed care may limit the number of visits, types of intervention, or conditions for approval of physical therapy. These cost-saving tactics also have been adopted by a variety of private insurers and workers' compensation programs, which means that PTs must consider financial factors when making decisions about their

Table 9-1 | **Organizational Terminology**

Term	Definition
Organization	A group that shares and pursues a common goal
System	Any group of interacting, interrelated, or interdependent parts that form a complex, unified whole with a specific purpose[4]
Organizational culture	The shared beliefs, values, symbols, acceptable behaviors, and rituals of an organization
Strategy	A plan or pattern of action for achieving the goals of an organization—it may be highly structured or more dynamic (emergent)—that is evolving rather than planned in advance[5]
Strategic planning	A planning process that involves evaluation of the organizational environment, goals, and objectives; analysis of the effect of specific situations on the goals and objectives; and a plan for the use of resources[5]
Leader	A person who influences or attempts to influence action, strategy, the organization's internal or external environment, or the organizational culture[5] (a variety of theories define leadership in terms of traits, behavior, reaction to situations, use of power and influence, fit between leader and situation, or other criteria[6])
Learning organization	A term used by Peter Senge[7] to describe an organization in which employees engage in ongoing learning so as to achieve a collective vision by practicing the five disciplines of the learning organization

patients. These day-to-day realities highlight two characteristics of the current health care system in the United States:

1. The health care "system" is not a single entity but a fragmented system made up of numerous smaller systems, including federal (Medicare), state (Medicaid), and local health care organizations (hospitals, insurance companies, private companies, equipment and drug manufacturers, and professional associations), as well as health care providers.[10]
2. The bureaucratic organizational model cannot be adapted to a system of this complexity.[3]

Anderson and McDaniel[3] point out that the "default" mental image of an organization tends to be one of a hierarchical bureaucracy with a rigidly defined chain of command that operates according to traditional administrative rules. However, several authors[11-14] have noted dysfunctional patterns that may develop in bureaucratically organized structures, including a tendency to focus on strict role delineation, displacement of the organizational mission in favor of mere survival, competition between subunits, overconformity in thought (i.e., "groupthink")[14] and behavior, a tendency to become a closed system that is out of touch with the outside environment, and numerous ill effects on communication and worker morale as a result of rigid hierarchical controls. For example, workers who find that their perspective is seldom acknowledged in decisions may rely on routine protocols without critical evaluation, and they may also stop communicating their concerns to middle and top management.

Anderson and McDaniel[3] suggest that the demands of the health care environment require a new organizational model, the *complex adaptive system.* Such an organization defines itself more in terms of relationships, feedback loops, synergy (the whole is greater than the sum of its parts) of the system's development. From this perspective, no one person has all of the knowledge necessary to direct the future of the organization. This organizational model requires skills for staff-level therapists and leaders that are different from those used in a professional bureaucracy.

Anderson and McDaniel[3] contrast the challenges of leadership in a bureaucracy with those encountered in a complex adaptive system (Box 9-1). In a bureaucracy, management must define problems, determine a course of action, and then tell others down the chain of command what to do. In a complex adaptive system, rarely can any one person make a determination about the entire system; therefore the fundamental task of the leader is to create a *learning organization* (see Table 9-1).[3] A learning organization accommodates the "unknowability" of the complex adaptive system, because employees engage in continual learning to achieve a collective vision. Senge[7] listed five disciplines for a learning organization: personal mastery, mental models, building a shared vision, team learning, and systems thinking.

Teams are the fundamental learning unit of the organization[7]; therefore team building and leadership become critical skills for PTs as contemporary health care moves from a bureaucracy model to a learning organization model. Through shared, team-based decision making, shared power, and continual efforts by employees to learn about the internal and external environment, learning organizations may avoid the organizational failings of bureaucracies.

THE IMPORTANCE OF ORGANIZATIONS AND SYSTEMS KNOWLEDGE

A health care organization's ability to evaluate changes in the health care system and mount an organizational response is an important survival tool. However, PTs' professional education may not give them experience and expertise in these important skills.[2] The challenge for educators, then, is to determine how to graduate PTs with these skills so that physical therapy as a profession has a greater impact on health care organizations and systems.

THE INDIVIDUAL, INSTITUTIONAL, AND SOCIETAL REALMS OF HEALTH CARE

To help practitioners deal with the inherent complexity of the current health care system, Glaser[1,15-17] has described health care as having three realms: the individual realm, the institutional (or organizational) realm, and the societal realm (Figure 9-1).

Box 9-1   **KEY LEADERSHIP TASKS IN A COMPLEX ADAPTIVE SYSTEM AND A PROFESSIONAL BUREAUCRACY**

Complex Adaptive System	Professional Bureaucracy
Relationship building	Role defining
Loose coupling	Creating a tight organizational structure
Complicating	Simplifying
Diversifying	Socializing to the organization
Sense making	Decision making
Learning	Knowing
Improvising	Controlling
Thinking about the future	Planning based on forecasting

Modified from Anderson RA, McDaniel RR Jr. Managing health care organizations: Where professionalism meets complexity science. *Health Care Manage Rev* 2000;25(1):83-92

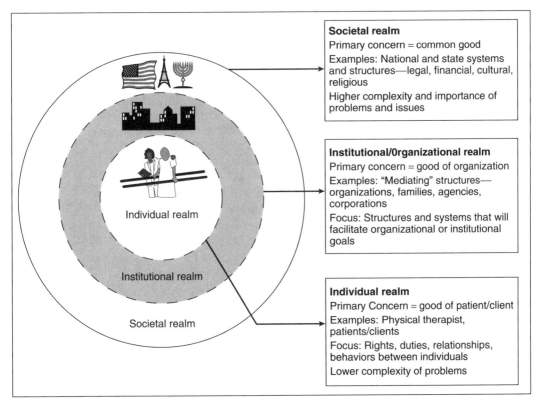

Figure 9-1. Glaser's three realms of health care. *(Modified from Glaser JW.* Three realms of ethics: Individual, institutional, societal. *Kansas City, Mo: Rowman & Littlefield; 1994.)*

This framework has its foundation in the individual and social natures of human reality, as well as the increasing level of complexity of the problems encountered by individuals, organizations, and society.[1,15-17] The three realms are interdependent and "nested" within one another; that is, every problem has an individual, an organizational, and a societal dimension, as well as an aspect Glaser calls a "cardinal realm,"[1,15-17] the critical realm for that particular issue. For example, the cardinal realm for the problem of justice in the allocation of health care resources exists at the societal level, and the cardinal realm for informed consent exists at the individual level. Even so, parts of both these problems belong to the other realms.

Glaser makes two other important points.[1,15-17] First, problems increase in complexity as they move from the individual to the societal realm. Problems are more complicated at the organizational level than at the individual level and are still more complex at the societal level. Second, deficits at one level cannot be offset at another level. Therefore the efforts of individual health care providers cannot make up for unfair societal health care arrangements (e.g., lack of health care insurance), and society cannot compensate for defects at the individual level (e.g., federal and state regulations covering informed consent and patient privacy are ineffective unless practitioners are ethical and establish trustworthy professional relationships).

The three-realm model of health care can be helpful to the PT in negotiating the complexity of the health care environment because it requires examination of the multiple levels of any problem.[1,15-17] Understanding the interrelationship of the three realms may help PTs understand the complexity of the issues involved across the spectrum of their professional decisions. For example, PTs may need to determine whether efficient, effective care can be provided within the constraints of available funding or whether they should support the legislative agenda of their professional organization. The ability to see the relationship between the inadequacy of the current health care system and the need to participate in efforts to change the system is critical if a PT is to function effectively in the changing health care environment.

In addition to Glaser's three realms, the PT must recognize the need to address cultural issues that influence every level of the health care system.

THE ROLE OF CULTURE IN HEALTH CARE

The population of the United States is becoming ever more diverse. The U.S. Census Bureau predicted that by the year 2005, minorities would account for half the population.[18] This increasing diversity has made it increasingly important that PTs understand cultural differences.

The term *culture* refers to the beliefs, attitudes, values, worldview, and patterns of behavior of a particular group of people. Race may contribute to a culture, but the words *race* and *culture* are not synonymous. In addition to physical attributes culture embraces behavior and attitudes, such as language, food preferences, style of dress, symbols, morality, rituals, and religious views. Culture is not monolithic; numerous, overlapping cultures may act on an individual simultaneously. Much of a culture is learned subconsciously, but a person may accept or reject values, beliefs, and behaviors.

Like nations, religions, and communities, organizations may have unique cultures, which include values, language, symbols, rituals, rites, and acceptable behaviors. Organizations have dominant cultures and subcultures. For example, a physical therapy department's subculture may be very different from the organizational culture of the hospital in which it is located.

Individual Cultural Competence

As professionals, PTs are expected to respect cultural differences and to incorporate an understanding of culture into patient/client management. The ability to recognize and respond appropriately to cultural differences is known as *cultural competence.*

As with clinical competence or professionalism, cultural competence develops throughout professional life. Cross[19,20] described cultural competence as a process on a continuum (Figure 9-2) that extends from the negative state of cultural destructiveness to cultural proficiency (Table 9-2).[19-23]

To become culturally proficient, an individual must acquire skills and knowledge that come from interacting with people of different backgrounds or cultures. Through the Internet and in textbooks, professionals can find numerous sources of information on improving communication and clinical intervention in intercultural situations. For the most part, this kind of information is either general or culture-specific. General information includes general principles and questions professionals can ask whenever they are dealing with a patient from another culture. Culture-specific information is detailed information about particular cultures. In reality, PTs need both approaches. Because a person cannot be knowledgeable about every culture and because individuals appropriate only part of their culture of origin, a general approach is necessary for negotiating cultural interactions. On the other hand, a knowledge of specific cultures is essential in many cases. Cultural evaluation of patients is a skill that every PT must have (Box 9-2).

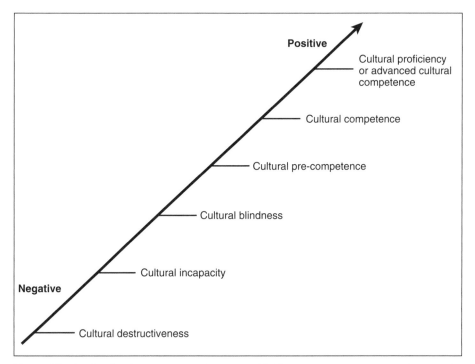

Figure 9-2. Cross's cultural competence continuum. (*Modified from Cross TL, Bazron BJ, Dennis KW, et al. Towards a culturally competent system of care: A monograph on effective services for minority children who are severely emotionally disturbed. Washington, DC: Georgetown University, Child Development Center; 1989.*)

Cultural Competence in the Organization

Cross's model of cultural competence can be applied to organizations as well as individuals.[19,20] An individual's cultural competence can be demonstrated through the methods of communication used, interactions with those of other cultures, and the extent to which relevant knowledge is incorporated into patient/client management. Evaluation of an organization's cultural competence focuses on hiring patterns, formal and informal policies for handling cultural conflict, inclusion of relevant groups in the decision-making process, and advocacy for minority groups. Mak[21] observed that the degree of cultural competence may vary, depending on the particular culture addressed by the individual or organization. For example, in race relations, an organization may be at the proficiency level, whereas in sexual orientation issues, it may be at the cultural destructiveness level.

Evaluating Cultural Competence

Glaser's three-realm model is congruent with Cross's suggestion that both individuals and organizations should be evaluated for cultural competence. Glaser's model pushes practitioners to ask themselves three questions:
1. What must I do to deliver culturally appropriate care?
2. What policies and procedures must be in place for the organization to promote cultural proficiency?
3. What national laws and policies are required to promote cultural proficiency?

Table 9-2 | **Levels of Culture Competence**

Level	Hallmarks
Cultural destructiveness	Individuals or organizations may view another culture as problematic or may encourage those of that culture to act more like the majority; destruction of minority cultures is actively sought.
Cultural incapacity	Individuals or organizations believe in the superiority of the mainstream culture but do not actively seek destruction of other cultures; stereotypes and paternalism are reinforced.
Cultural blindness	Individuals or organizations treat everyone the same, without regard for culture (implicitly reinforce the dominant culture).
Cultural precompetence	Individuals or organizations recognize cultural differences, as well as their weaknesses in addressing them, and seek to become educated about these differences.
Cultural competence	Individuals or organizations respect cultural differences, make changes to accommodate these differences, and engage in analysis of cultural interactions.
Cultural proficiency	Individuals or organizations hold cultural differences in high regard, educate others and develop skills in addressing such differences, and partner with those of other cultures.

Modified from Cross TL, Bazron BJ, Dennis KW, et al. Towards a culturally competent system of care: A monograph on effective services for minority children who are severely emotionally disturbed. Vol 1. Washington, DC: Georgetown University Child Development Center; 1989.

The models of Cross and Glaser also reinforce the distinction between individual prejudice and "institutional bias" or discrimination.

LEADERSHIP AND PHYSICAL THERAPY

Although most would agree that leaders are important in organizations, scholars disagree over whether leaders are defined by personal traits, power, or the ability to influence others, behaviors, or actions. A distinction is often made between leadership and management because a manager may simply be an individual designated to hold a position of authority and provide administrative oversight. From this standpoint, one need not be a manager to be a leader. As discussed previously, Anderson and McDaniel[3] contend that complex adaptive systems require leadership skills radically different from those needed in bureaucratic organizations (see Box 9-1 and Table 8-1).

PTs serve as leaders in other areas besides health care organizations. They participate in professional organizations, such as the American Physical Therapy Association (APTA); they help in the local community; they serve as members of boards and agencies; and they participate in local, state, and national politics. If Glaser's three-realm model is applied to the concept of leadership, PTs would seem obligated to be leaders only in the development of health care policies. Because societal problems cannot be remediated at the organizational and individual levels, PTs must exercise leadership in the political arena to achieve the goal of fair health care laws and policies.

Box **9-2**   **CONSIDERATIONS IN THE CULTURAL EVALUATION OF PATIENTS**

Leininger's Sunrise Model*

- Cultural values and ways of living
- Religious, philosophical, and spiritual beliefs
- Economic factors
- Educational factors
- Attitudes toward technology
- Kinship and social ties
- Political and legal factors

Davidhizar, Bechtel, and Giger Model†

- Communication
- Space
- Time
- Social organization
- Environmental control
- Biological variations

Modified from U.S. Department of Health and Human Services, Office of Minority Health. *Stage II: Conceptualizing cultural competence and identifying critical domains.* Retrieved April 16, 2004, at http://www.hrsa.gov/OMH/cultural/sectionii.htm#A.%20%20%20%20%20Approaches%20to%20conceptualizing%20cultural%20competence
*Leininger M. Towards conceptualization of a transcultural health care system: Concepts and a model. *J Transcult Nurs* 1993;4(2):32-40.
†Davidhizar R, Bechtel G, Giger JN. A model to enhance culturally competent care. *Hosp Top* 1998;76(2): 22-26.

A FOURTH REALM: THE INTERNATIONAL

Glaser's concept could be extended to include a fourth realm, the international realm. Information systems, globalization, environmental concerns, and economics increasingly are bringing together all parts of the world. However, individuals find it more difficult to conceptualize international connections than organizational or national systems. As Glaser's model shows, problems at this level are extraordinarily complex because they involve diverse nations, governmental systems, ethnic histories, and cultures. In addition, different countries have different beliefs about the meaning of health; they also have different health care reimbursement systems and varying technological and financial support of health care services.

Given these national and regional differences, the tremendous variation in the provision of physical therapy around the world is not surprising. In some areas physical therapy practice is similar to that seen in the United States during the 1970s or 1980s. In Canada, the United Kingdom, and western Europe, the practice of physical therapy is somewhat similar to that in the United States except for the reimbursement system. In contrast to the United States, most of the western developed nations have a single-payer system in which the government pays for a large part of health care.

The extended four-realm version of Glaser's model suggests that PTs should be interested in physical therapy in other countries. Dialog with PTs in other countries has the potential to enrich all participants.

FURTHER THOUGHTS

PTs do not practice in a vacuum. Indeed, the work of the PT not only is located within organizational, social, cultural, and political contexts but also demands skills in using resources from these contexts to the benefit of patients from diverse backgounds. Many PTs are attracted to the profession by the opportunity to work closely with individual patients and may have negative preconceptions about negotiating the organizational and social realms. In addition, PTs may view organizations through the lens of the old bureaucratic models. Undoubtedly, one of the most important lessons of managed care is the importance of organizations and health care systems in the delivery of health care in the United States. Acquiring and maintaining knowledge and skills relevant to building effective health care organizations and systems and negotiating across cultures is an important element of professionalism for individuals and organizations. As the United States continues to struggle with rising health care costs and increasing diversity, these skills will become even more important for PTs.

CASE SCENARIOS

Case Scenario 1

You accept a new job as supervisor of the outpatient area in a local hospital. After finishing your first week, you decide that you like the work and your colleagues. However, you are concerned about several comments about race and religion made over the course of the week that seemed to reflect a lack of cultural competence and even to show bias.
- *Use Cross's framework to evaluate the cultural competence of the individuals concerned.*
- *How can you facilitate cultural competence?*
- *What can you do to change the organizational culture?*

Case Scenario 2

Mohammed was treated for 6 weeks in the physical therapy department of St. Ignatius Hospital for rehabilitation of a rotator cuff injury. Your co-worker, Jonathan, was able to help him regain his former level of function although Jonathan once confided to you over lunch that Mohammed made him "nervous." Two weeks after Mohammed was discharged, a patient satisfaction survey arrived by mail stating that "the physical therapy department discriminates against Muslims." Nobody can remember any specific incident, but the assumption is that the complaint came from Mohammed.
- *As head of the physical therapy department, how would you handle the complaint?*
- *How would you evaluate the cultural competence of your department and your organization?*

Case Scenario 3

Three visits for physical therapy have been authorized for your patient, Mr. Smith. You begin your plan of care knowing that three visits will not be enough to enable Mr. Smith to achieve the goals that would allow him to live alone in his home safely. Your supervisor tells you that the hospital's policy is not to request authorization from Mr. Smith's insurance company because "they always say no."
- *What do you do? (Use Glaser's three realms to analyze your decision.)*

QUESTIONS FOR REFLECTION

1. What does the term *leader* mean to you? Think of an important leader in your life; why do you think of that person as a leader? How does the leader differ from the manager?

2. In making career choices, how will you determine whether a health care organization is a bureaucracy or a learning organization? What difference does it make to your work as a professional?

3. How would you evaluate your own cultural competence in general and with regard to specific issues of race, gender, sexual orientation, and religion? Use Cross's continuum to indicate your own cultural competence and that of your organization, the profession, and society. (Use an *X* for yourself, an *O* for your organization, a *P* for the profession, and an *S* for society).

4. Ruth Purtilo[24] has argued that physical therapists should be involved in the formulation of health care policy. Do physical therapists have an obligation to participate in the political process? Why or why not?

5. The United States has been criticized as having lack of access to and inequities in the distribution of health care resources. Would you support the development of a single-payer system? How would this affect each of Glaser's realms of health care?

6. Review the discussion of the Health Insurance Portability and Accountability Act (HIPAA) in Chapter 8. Which of Glaser's three realms does this legislation address? How should privacy be protected in each realm?

7. It could be argued that including the family in rehabilitation planning is different from considering family systems issues. What would it mean to consider the family as a system, as Glaser's model suggests? How would this influence patient/client management?

REFERENCES

1. Glaser JW, Hamel RP. Introduction. In Glaser JW, Hamel RP, editors. *Three realms of managed care: Societal, institutional, individual.* Kansas City, Mo: Sheed & Ward; 1997.

2. Lopopolo RB, Schafer DS, Nosse LJ. Leadership, administration, management, and professionalism (LAMP) in physical therapy: A Delphi study. *Phys Ther* 2004;84(2):137-150.

3. Anderson RA, McDaniel RR Jr. Managing health care organizations: Where professionalism meets complexity science. *Health Care Manage Rev* 2000;25(1):83-92.

4. Kim DH. *Introduction to systems thinking.* Waltham, Mass: Pegasus; 1999.

5. Mintzberg HM, Quinn JB, Voyer J. *The strategy process.* Englewood Cliffs, NJ: Prentice Hall; 1995.

6. Yukl G: *Leadership in organizations* (3rd ed). Englewood Cliffs, NJ: Prentice Hall; 1994.

7. Senge P. The fifth discipline: The art and practice of the learning organization. In Ott. SJ, editor. Classic readings in organizational behavior (2nd ed). Belmont, Calif: Wadsworth; 1996.

8. Caughey A, Sabin J. Managed care. In Calkins D, Fernandopulle RJ, Marino BS, editors. *Healthcare policy.* Cambridge, Mass: Blackwell Science; 1995.

9. Giffin A. Coping with the prospective payment system (PPS): Ethical issues in rehabilitation. *Issues on Aging* 2000;23(1):2-8.

10. Rothman DJ. *Strangers at the bedside: A history of how law and bioethics transformed medical decision making.* New York: Basic Books; 1991.

11. Merton RK. Bureaucratic structure and personality. In Ott SJ, editor. *Classic readings in organizational behavior* (2nd ed). Belmont, Calif: Wadsworth; 1996. pp.337-343.

12. March JG, Simon HA. Theories of bureaucracy. In Shafritz JM, Ott SJ, editors. *Classics of organization theory* (3rd ed). Belmont, Calif: Wadsworth; 1992. pp. 124-132.

13. Mintzberg HM. *Professional bureaucracy.* Retrieved at www.lib.usf.edu/ereserve/EDH7636001/Z.pdf

14. Janis IL. Groupthink: The desperate drive for consensus at any cost. In Ott SJ, editor. *Classic readings in organizational behavior* (2nd ed). Belmont, Calif: Wadsworth; 1996.

15. Glaser JW. Phase II of bioethics: The turn to the social nature of individuals. Bioethics Forum 1995;Fall.

16. Glaser JW, Glaser BB. Systemic reform is vital to our ministry. *Health Progress* 2002;May-June: 16-19.

17. Glaser JW. *Three realms of ethics: Individual, institutional, societal.* Kansas City, Mo: Sheed & Ward; 1994.

18. US Census Bureau. Retrieved April 14, 2004, at http://www.census.gov/ipc/www/usinterimproj

19. Cross TL, Bazron BJ, Dennis KW, et al. *Towards a culturally competent system of care: A monograph on effective services for minority children who are severely emotionally disturbed.* Vol 1. Washington, DC: Georgetown University; Child Development Center; 1989.

20. Cross TL. *Cultural competence continuum.* Retrieved April 16, 2004, at http://www.nysccc.org/T0Rarts/ CultCompCont.html

21. Mak J. *What is cultural competency?* Retrieved April 16, 2004, at http://lanecc.edu/afirmact/dhrc/docs/cultural_comp.pdf

22. Washington State Department of Health, Multicultural Work Group. *Building cultural competence.* Retrieved April 16, 2004, at http://www.doh.wa.gov/cfh/Pubs/MCWG2001Lo.pdf

23. US Department of Health and Human Services, Office of Minority Health. *Stage II: Conceptualizing cultural competence and identifying critical domains.* Retrieved April 16, 2004, at http://www.hrsa.gov/OMH/cultural/sectionii.htm#A.%20%20%20%20%20Approaches%20to%20conceptualizing%20cultural%20competence

24. Purtilo RB. Who should make moral policy decisions in health care? *Phys Ther* 1978;58:1076-1081.

Professional Development, Competence, and Expertise

Throughout a professional career, professionals will be changing the scope of their competence, through becoming more specialist, through moving into newly developing areas of professional work, or through taking on management or educational roles; they will also be continuously developing the quality of their work in a number of areas, beyond the level of competence to one of proficiency or expertise.

– Michael Eraut[1]

Where are the standards for CE [continuing education]? If you find them, let me know—and let me know how they are implemented and by whom. In states that require CE units (CEUs) for physical therapists to maintain their licenses, there is a patchwork of mechanisms for CEU approval, almost none of which are related to the quality of the content. In many of those states, we use CEUs to argue with legislators that we are policing our own house and that we are as professional as anyone else. But that masks the reality. Our argument implies that we are doing something to protect the public, when in fact we are doing something for self-aggrandizement and political purposes and to keep the CE industry incredibly profitable. Unless we do something to ensure that CE courses are based on recent, credible information, we aren't helping patients.

–Jules Rothstein[2]

THE LIFELONG PROCESS OF SKILL ENHANCEMENT

Although professionals spend years acquiring an education to prepare themselves for their roles, professional education is merely the first step toward attaining the knowledge and skills needed to practice. The constant expansion of knowledge and technological innovation in health care demand that physical therapists (PTs) and other professionals engage in a lifelong process of enhancing their professional knowledge and skills.

Most would agree that practitioners have an obligation to maintain professional competency, although there is considerably less agreement on what this process entails or how it should be evaluated. Nevertheless, concern about incompetent practitioners has made professional development and continued competence important public issues. The following questions reflect some of the concerns about professional development and competence:

1. What is professional development, and how should it be measured?
2. How should clinical competence be assessed? Should it be determined by the number of continuing education units (CEUs) acquired, periodic reexamination, self-assessment, peer review, licensure, or some combination of these methods?
3. Who should evaluate the competence of a PT or physical therapist assistant (PTA)—members of the profession, state licensing boards, employing organizations, peers, or the individual practitioner?
4. How is professional competence different from professional development?
5. What responsibility should the profession take for identifying incompetent PTs and preventing them from practicing?
6. How should PTs approach professional development? What resources are available to assist in professional development?
7. How can a PT use a portfolio in the professional development process?

This chapter provides a definition of professional development, distinguishes professional competence from professional development or career success, explores activities in professional development, discusses the background of and controversies in professional development, presents the perspectives of different involved groups on professional development, and provides some strategies for the professional development process

THE PROFESSIONAL DEVELOPMENT CONTINUUM: FROM COMPETENCE TO EXPERTISE

Two primary elements of professionalism are specialized skills and training. Professional skills are dynamic and contextual; clinical approaches change based on emerging research, and they may be applied differently in different organizations or practice settings. Professionals have some autonomy in applying their professional skills and knowledge, but through the implied contract with society, they have an obligation to protect the public from incompetent practitioners and to improve their skills continuously so as to best meet the needs of their patients.

As professionals, PTs also have an obligation to update their skills. The *Guide for Professional Conduct* (GPC) of the American Physical Therapy Association (APTA) takes note of this: "A physical therapist has a lifelong professional responsibility for maintaining competence through ongoing self-assessment, education, and enhancement of knowledge and skills" (GPC 5.2).[3]

Some might refer to this simply as maintaining continued competency to practice, but maintaining minimal clinical competency is only part of the professional development process. The APTA statement on professional development (Box 10-1) incorporates many of the somewhat conflicting aspects of the process: maintenance of minimal competence, lifelong learning, and adaptation to the challenges posed by organizations, the various contexts of health care, and the PT's chosen career path.[4]

Scope of Competence

Eraut[1] notes that competence and professional development have very different connotations. Competence suggests a dichotomous evaluation; that is, a person is either competent or not to perform a particular task. Professional development is more

Professional development encompasses the entire scope of a career, beginning with preprofessional education and continuing throughout the professional life span. Professional development enables individuals who work in the profession of physical therapy to assume an attitude of inquiry and to engage in assessment and actions that will provide the opportunity to (1) maintain and update knowledge and skills; (2) achieve induction into new responsibility; (3) recapture the mastery of concepts; and (4) create, anticipate, and actively respond to change.

Each member is obligated to participate in professional development to ensure the acquisition and maintenance of minimally acceptable standards of practice. Every individual has the right to engage in professional development based on attitude, assessment, and need at a preferred level exceeding acceptable standards of practice.

Professional development may occur in formal instructional settings or in natural societal settings and may include such varied experiences as academic courses of study, organized continuing education, independent study, and self- and external assessment. The variety of experiences may be as diverse as the sponsors, content, and teaching and learning styles of those participating. The APTA has the responsibility to interpret the concepts and scope of professional development in a manner consistent with the APTA objectives, functions, and strategic planning process. The concepts and scope of professional development will be translated into appropriate activities that are responsive to the current and future needs of members, the organization, and the profession.

consistent with evaluation on a continuous scale ranging from novice to expert (Figures 10-1 and 10-2). Professional development connotes a process of continuous improvement, lifelong learning, and growth, which allow professionals to improve their practice so as to better serve patients, clients, organizations, the profession, and society.[1]

Eraut[1] describes two dimensions of professional competence: scope and quality. The *scope of competence* includes the roles, tasks, and skills a professional can perform and the situations or circumstances in which they can be performed. For example, a PT or PT student who demonstrates competence in joint mobilization while using a simulated orthopedic patient in a classroom setting may not have

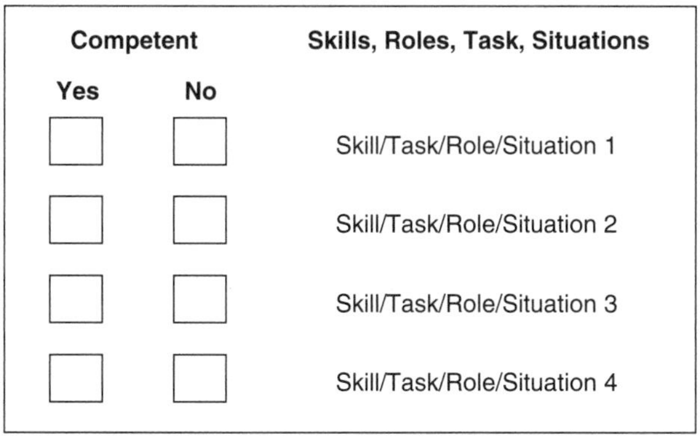

Figure 10-1. Scope of professional competence. *(Modified from Eraut M. Developing professional knowledge and competence. London: Falmer; 1994.)*

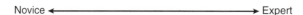

Figure 10-2. Quality of professional competence. *(Modified from Eraut M. Developing professional knowledge and competence. London: Falmer; 1994.)*

similar competence in the clinical setting or with patients with neurological diagnoses. The student's scope of competence, therefore, is more limited than that of the expert manual therapist, who has had more opportunity to perform the skill in a variety of circumstances.

Quality

Whereas the scope of competence focuses on whether or not a professional is able to perform tasks under various circumstances,[1] the dimension of *quality* addresses how well the professional performs these tasks. Some skills, such as communication of basic information, do not necessarily depend on quality for effectiveness; other skills, such as spinal joint mobilization, have a very narrow scope of competence but require high quality to be effective.[1] Meaningful professional development seeks to enhance both dimensions of competence—scope and quality.

By considering both dimensions of professional competence, PTs and PTAs may think beyond the focus on technical skills, the commonly accepted perspective of competence. Although most professionals pursue opportunities in professional development to enhance their technical capabilities, Eraut's model suggests that professional expertise involves much more than hands-on skills.

Expertise

Epstein and Hundert[5] define professional competence in the medical context as "the habitual and judicious use of communication, knowledge, technical skills, clinical reasoning, emotions, values, and reflection in daily practice for the benefit of the individual and community being served."

In addition to technical skills, expertise in physical therapy involves a blending of cognitive, technical, psychosocial, interactive, and moral skills.[5] In a qualitative study of expertise in four specialty areas of physical therapy, Jensen and colleagues[6] identified four dimensions of clinical expertise (Figure 10-3):

1. Multidimensional, patient-centered knowledge base that evolves through reflection
2. Collaborative and problem-solving approach to clinical reasoning
3. Focus on movement linked to patient function
4. Sense of caring and commitment to patients

Whereas Jensen et al[6] found PTs regarded by their peers as experts and looked for common dimensions, other research has examined expertise on the basis of clinical outcomes. Resnik and Jensen[7] compared the characteristics of "expert" and "average" PTs on the basis of clinical outcomes achieved with patients (Table 10-1). PTs who achieved superior outcomes ("experts") used a patient-centered approach, one founded on caring and respect and directed toward patient empowerment. Unlike the average PTs, the expert practitioners also had a broader knowledge base that integrated previous experiences and peer consultation, were humble in recognizing their limitations, reflected on their practice, and expressed a passion for clinical practice.[7]

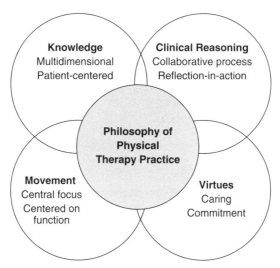

Figure 10-3.   Four dimensions of clinical expertise in physical therapy. *(From Jensen GM, Gwyer J, Shepard KF et al. Expert practice in physical therapy.* Phys Ther *2000;80[1]:28-43.)*

An interesting finding emerged from this study: specialty education, clinical experience, commitment to professional growth, and opportunities for growth were not distinguishing factors between expert and average PTs.[7] This would seem to suggest that education and opportunity may be "necessary but not sufficient" factors in professional expertise.

The practical significance of the models and attributes of expertise discussed in this section is fourfold:

1.   Professional development requires activities involving all four dimensions of practice: (i.e., a multidimensional knowledge base, a collaborative problem-solving approach to clinical reasoning, a focus on movement linked to patient function, and a sense of caring and commitment toward patients).

2.   The development of professional expertise also requires cultivation of attributes and behaviors such as humility, passion for clinical work, collegial interaction, and limited delegation to support staff.

3.   Professional competence is dynamic, changing constantly in relation to organizational and contextual roles.

4.   Physical therapists must assess their skills in the numerous dimensions of professional expertise and seek professional development in all dimensions, attributes, and behaviors throughout their careers. In addition to continuing education courses that focus on knowledge and clinical reasoning, PTs should seek opportunities to enhance their personal growth and interactive skills.

ACTIVITIES THAT PROMOTE PROFESSIONAL DEVELOPMENT

Many activities may promote professional development (Box 10-2). Although the list in Box 10-2 is not exhaustive, it shows the diversity of activities that may contribute to the development of professional expertise in physical therapy.

Table 10-1 | **Attributes of Expert and Average Physical Therapists**

Categories	Expert	Average
Clinical Reasoning		
1. Patient empowerment a primary goal of therapy	✓	
2. Collaborative problem-solving approach	✓	
3. Context of clinical practice: teacher/coach	✓	
Knowledge Base		
1. Eclectic academic background	✓	
2. Undergraduate degrees in exercise science	✓	
3. Field experience prior to physical therapy school	✓	
4. Frequent use of collegial knowledge	✓	
5. Greater use of movement observation	✓	
6. Reflection on practice	✓	
7. Extent of clinical experience	✓	✓
8. Specialty knowledge from continuing education	✓	✓
9. Knowledge from patients	✓	✓
10. History as a patient receiving physical therapy	✓	✓
11. Athletic background	✓	✓
Values and Virtues		
1. Love of clinical care	✓	
2. Humility	✓	
3. Inquisitiveness	✓	
4. Caring	✓	✓
5. Commitment to professional growth	✓	✓
Clinical Practice Style		
1. Patient education central to practice	✓	
2. Individualized interventions	✓	
3. Limited delegation of care to support personnel	✓	
4. Extensive use of growth opportunities in the workplace	✓	✓

Modified from Resnik L, Jensen GM. Using clinical outcomes to explore the theory of expert practice in physical therapy. Phys Ther *2003;83:1090-1106.*

However, as Resnik and Jensen[7] found, participation in these activities does not automatically guarantee enhanced professional expertise and development. For example, those who attend continuing education courses sometimes find they are unable to use what they have learned in their clinical practice. This disconnection between teaching and learning may have several causes.

One cause may be that the course emphasizes formal knowledge over reflective knowledge. In describing reflective practice, Shepard and Jensen[8] built on the work of Schon,[9] which distinguished formal, or technical, knowledge from reflective, or intuitive, knowledge. In contrast to technical knowledge, which focuses on facts and rules, reflective knowledge incorporates the intuition used in everyday practice. Reflective knowledge allows the practitioner to solve the ill-defined clinical problems of everyday practice that do not match the standard rules and examples of formal knowledge; a practitioner with reflective knowledge "holds the knowledge and skills of a technical practitioner and is skilled in creative information acquisition and intervention techniques that can be brought to bear on any unique

Box 10-2   Activities that Promote Professional Development

- Formal continuing education courses
- Employer inservice or education opportunities
- Internship or residency practice
- Changes in work position and new challenges
- Individual research on topics of interest
- Reading professional journals
- Clinical experience
- Professional association activities
- Clinical specialization
- Journal clubs
- Career ladders (pathways that specify the competencies necessary for professional advancement)
- Interaction with colleagues
- Working with a mentor
- Peer review
- Self-assessment
- Postprofessional education
- Study groups
- Participation in interdisciplinary teams
- Participation in clinical research
- Leadership in professional associations
- Development of a professional portfolio
- Reflective practice

health care problem that may be encountered during the practice of physical therapy."[8]

A professional development activity also may fail to produce professional growth because the activity may not be an appropriate vehicle for meeting the learner's goals. For example, a PT who wants to become a skilled manual therapist may select a continuing education course for that purpose but may not have the opportunity to use the skills that are taught. Without this opportunity, the PT is unlikely to be able to apply the knowledge gained in the course. Similarly, a learner may select a course without having a real plan for practicing and refining the skills involved, or the person may chose a course simply because it is convenient or inexpensive.

The quality of the continuing education course is another factor that determines whether a professional development activity produces professional growth. In a poor-quality course, the instructional strategies may be inadequate, instruction may be offered at an introductory level, or the latest developments in the field may not be included in the course content. Although many states require continuing education, very few evaluate the quality of these courses; that responsibility rests primarily with the participants. The *Guide for Professional Conduct* urges PTs to use sound judgment in evaluating continuing education courses: "A physical therapist shall evaluate the efficacy and effectiveness of information and techniques presented in continuing education programs before integrating them into his or her practice" (GPC 6.4C).[3]

Failure of continuing education to foster professional expertise may also result from a lack of motivation on the part of the participant. If the PT's motivation is to fulfill a requirement rather than to enhance expertise, professional development may not result. For example, in states that require continuing education, licensees often select a course on the basis of expense or convenience rather than professional needs.

Because participation in professional development activities does not guarantee greater expertise, the issue becomes how to measure professional development and competence.

EVALUATION OF COMPETENCE AND PROFESSIONAL DEVELOPMENT

The initial licensure requirement ensures that the public is protected from unqualified individuals who try to enter a profession. The state regulatory boards, which are responsible for setting licensure standards, must therefore develop some mechanism for ensuring that those who apply for licensure and relicensure are competent to practice. Although these mechanisms may seem inconvenient, PTs and PTAs cannot avoid evaluation of professional competence.

As has been shown, professional development and professional competence are complex, multidimensional concepts. It is not surprising, therefore, that no agreement has been reached on how to evaluate them, and most efforts focus only on knowledge and skills rather than the expanded dimensions of competence. The following are four possible approaches to evaluation of professional competence in physical therapy:

- Mandatory continuing education[10]
- Reexamination at set intervals[10]
- Peer review
- Compilation of a professional portfolio

Each of these approaches emphasizes a different aspect of professional development or competence (Table 10-2).

Mandatory Continuing Education

Mandatory continuing education is the most common approach to ensuring continuing professional competence in the United States. Many states require that PTs

Table **10-2** **Comparison of Approaches to Professional Development**

Component	Mandatory Continuing Education	Relicensure	Peer Review	Portfolio
Ease of evaluation	High	Low	Varies	Low
Ease of administration	High	Low	Varies	Low
Cost	Varies	High	Low	High
Promotion of minimal competence	Moderate	High	Low	Varies
Promotion of quality/expertise	Low	Low	Varies	High
Protection of public from gross incompetence	Moderate	Moderate	Low	Varies
Incorporation of contextual factors	Low	Low	High	High
Promotion of reflective practice	Low	Low	Varies	High
Adaptability to health care environment	Low	Moderate	Moderate	High

and PTAs engage in continuing education. Some states require that the CEUs be obtained in specific subjects, such as state law, ethics, medical error, recognition of domestic violence, care of patients infected with the human immunodeficiency virus, and clinical practice. A study of PTs done in the 1980s found that most respondents preferred continuing education over periodic reexamination.[8]

Mandatory continuing education is a popular approach to professional development and one that may prompt unmotivated professionals to pursue additional learning; however, it is not guaranteed to contribute to competence, quality, or expertise. In fact, some evidence indicates that continuing education is relatively ineffective at promoting professional development.[2] Nevertheless, continuing education has the potential to include areas beyond skills and knowledge and to focus on expertise versus minimal competence.

Reexamination

Reexamination would require professionals to take a written or practical examination (or both) at specified intervals. For example, a state board might require all PTs to take the licensure examination every 5 years. This approach appears to have the advantage of evaluating each PT for minimal competence, but it does not necessarily promote quality or expertise.

An additional question is whether the examination for relicensure should be more rigorous than that for initial licensure. PTs with specialized knowledge and skills may not do well on a test of entry-level procedures, but they may be quite skilled at performing the advanced physical therapy techniques required for their expert roles. Furthermore, written or practical relicensure examinations may not actually test the kind of knowledge and skills used in physical therapy practice because of the difficulty of creating an exam that captures the breadth of knowledge and dynamic nature of clinical interactions. For example, a written exam can evaluate the ability to select a correct diagnosis but not the interaction skills needed to take an appropriate history. Testing all of the skills required of PTs would be impossible in a practical examination format.

For all these reasons, some have proposed alternative routes to the establishment of professional competence, such as requiring PTs either to pass a relicensure examination or to provide evidence of professional specialization.

Peer Review

In a peer review system, experienced PTs evaluate the performance of other PTs. Many organizations use peer review as part of a yearly evaluation process. A supervisor may review one or more cases or may observe the PT during an examination or intervention. A rigorous peer review process can provide excellent feedback that may serve as a basis for professional growth. However, the process often has limitations, such as the following:

- Performance criteria are not formally articulated.
- Peer reviewers are not trained in providing reliable assessments.
- Peer reviewers are not skilled in providing constructive feedback.
- The link between the evaluation results and compensation impedes rigorous evaluation because peer reviewers are reluctant to prevent employees from receiving raises.

- Organizational standards or needs conflict with or supercede professional criteria for performance (e.g., the peer review may be most concerned with efficiency or documentation that nets reimbursement).
- Concerns about teamwork prevent peer reviewers from being completely honest in their appraisals.
- No formal link exists between the review and professional growth or the needs of the organization; also, the organization's needs for professional development may not coincide with the person's needs.

Professional Portfolio Compilation

Just as an artist might compile a portfolio of paintings to demonstrate artistic capability, the PT may collect exemplars[11] or artifacts that provide evidence of continuing professional growth. Many of those who advocate the use of portfolios emphasize that continuing reflection by PTs on their practice is essential to the process.[11] From this perspective, the portfolio should not be "scripted" but rather should be based on the insights of the therapist and driven by that individual's unique goals for professional development.

However, if the goal of the evaluation process is to protect the public from incompetence, the portfolio may need to be more structured. Faculty members in many institutions, for example, are required to assemble a rather structured portfolio in the tenure review process. In most cases the institution specifies the contents, although some latitude is allowed in the presentation of individual documents. Portfolios may serve many purposes, and the goals and outcomes for the portfolio must be specified at the outset (see Professional Development Planning section).

PROFESSIONAL DEVELOPMENT PLANNING

For many PTs the data from each of these evaluation tools can be combined to create a strategy for professional development. However, none of these efforts will be meaningful unless the PT reflects on the meaning of the items in the portfolio as they relate to the plan for professional development.

The Goal-Driven Portfolio

As noted previously, a professional portfolio is a tool PTs and other professionals can use to organize the many components of professional development. Paschal, Jensen, and Mostrom[11] created an outline for the portfolio used by students in the transitional doctor of physical therapy degree program at Creighton University. It includes the following:

1. A mission statement
2. A self-assessment
3. Exemplars supporting the self-assessment
4. A reflective analysis of the self-assessment (What? So what? Now what?)
5. A statement of goals
6. Plans for building strengths and addressing weaknesses

The professional development portfolio is both product and process.[11] As product, it is a tangible compilation of evidence of professional development. However, it would have no importance without the process of reflection and planning that resulted in its compilation.

The Process of Reflection and Planning

To begin the process of compiling a portfolio, the PT should compose an individual professional mission statement. The mission statement defines the therapist in terms of competencies and focuses on what the individual is currently doing while identifying resources for further development. The mission statement should be clear, concise, meaningful, easy to remember, accurate, dynamic, powerful, and focused.

The next step, self-assessment, is the heart of the process. In the self-assessment, the PT identifies strengths and weaknesses in relation to the personal mission. One approach to self-assessment is a strengths-weaknesses-opportunities-threats (SWOT) analysis,[12] in which the PT evaluates strengths and weaknesses (which are internal characteristics) and opportunities and threats (which are external factors). Self-assessment also may include input from peers and colleagues familiar with the PT's work.

For PTs, a vision statement reflects what they want to become and how they want to influence the world around them; it defines the individual's goals and values. It also is a clear, concise, meaningful statement of where the PT will be at some point in the future, such as 5 years from now. This process is aided by inclusion of exemplars or artifacts that support the self-assessment, such as continuing education certificates, written evaluations, and journal publications.

Reflection on the self-assessment is an important step, because the PT must determine what the honest self-assessment indicates.

In the final steps, the therapist should reexamine goals and make specific plans for building strengths and addressing weaknesses. Implementation of these plans should bring the PT back to reflection on the mission statement and self-assessment, creating a continuous cycle of planning and reflection.

Other approaches can be taken to pursue professional development; the process of self-assessment and goal setting may be more important than a product that reflects that process. However, a professional portfolio may become an important resource for future employment and career choices. Portfolios also may serve as a means of addressing the issues related to evaluation of competence.

POSSIBLE EVALUATORS OF PROFESSIONAL ACHIEVEMENT

Another important issue related to evaluation of professional competence and development is the determination of who should be responsible for this process: regulatory and licensing agencies, professional associations, employing organizations, or individual professionals?

In considering this question, it is helpful to take the perspective of each of these stakeholders:

- Many PTs believe that, as professionals, they are ultimately responsible for determining the activities and knowledge they need to maintain competence. In reality, each stakeholder plays a role in the evaluation of professional competence.
- Some argue that because regulatory and licensing agencies are charged by the state with protecting the public from incompetent or impaired practitioners, these agencies should be responsible for evaluation.
- Professional organizations may contend that they alone have the expertise and knowledge to evaluate professional competence. Because of the special

knowledge and expertise required by professional status, it may be argued that the profession itself, through its representative organization, should establish criteria for competence. Advocates of professional autonomy may also contend that professional status includes the obligation and privilege of self-regulation. Professionals typically participate in evaluation of professional competence by sitting on state licensing boards. In addition, in many states the state chapter of the APTA approves or accredits continuing education courses. However, some on state licensing boards may believe that physical therapists have been ineffective at self-regulation.

- Employing organizations may take the position that only they understand the unique contextual application of the knowledge the professional will use and that the organization bears the legal and financial burden of a PT's lack of competence. In this regard, mandatory organizational educational requirements (e.g., cardiopulmonary resuscitation, standard precautions) also determine professional competence.

A related question is who should pay for continuing education. When PTs were in short supply, employers provided money for continuing education as a benefit. However, with the increase in the number of physical therapists, as well as the financial pressure on health care organizations, many PTs are paying for professional development activities themselves. When the organization pays for continuing education, the PT may be expected to select an activity or course that directly enhances the skills used in the therapist's current position.

Regardless of the actions and demands of other stakeholders, each PT must take responsibility for professional development and commit to a planned approach that embraces the numerous dimensions of professional competence. Professional development that strives for maximum expertise rather than minimal competence benefits individual patients, society as a whole, and the profession. Ideally, this process is a lifelong journey of continuing efforts to enhance professional skills and knowledge. It requires commitment, honest self-assessment, reflection, and the input of peers, patients, and the professional organization.

CAREER ADVANCEMENT

The terms *career* and *career success* are closely related to professional development. However, the two terms are subtly different. The *Merriam-Webster Online Dictionary*[13] defines a *career* as "[the] pursuit of consecutive progressive achievement, especially in public, professional, or business life."[13] This definition suggests a *pattern* of achievement or success. Rozier and associates[14] defined *career success* as "the perception of an individual's employment achievements over time." Although professional development emphasizes the process of continuous education and improvement in skills, career advancement focuses more on professional success as measured by promotions, salary increases, enhancement of one's reputation, and other personal indicators of success.

A recurring question is whether men and women travel different gender-related paths in career advancement. For example, some professionals consider promotion an indicator of career success. However, women historically have had difficulty winning promotions because of a "glass ceiling" (an intangible barrier that prevents the promotion of women, primarily because of their sex, to the very top positions in the organization). Although it seems counterintuitive, women in female-dominated professions may also have difficulty achieving promotion to the highest levels. A study by Kemp and colleagues[15] in 1979 found that male PTs were more likely to be self-employed, hold more supervisory positions, and have higher incomes than female PTs. In 1998 Rozier and associates[14] noted that figures compiled by the APTA continued to show that female PTs earned less in salary and benefits, held fewer leadership positions, owned fewer private practices, and attained proportionately fewer clinical specializations than their male counterparts.

Other differences in the career paths of men and women in physical therapy also appear to exist. A study of PTs' perceptions of career success demonstrated that PTs defined career success somewhat differently from other professionals.[14] Both male and female PTs defined it more in terms of internal indicators (ethical practice, improving the health of the patient, personal satisfaction, and personal goals) than external factors (high income, administrative status). However, family responsibilities played a much greater role in women's concept of career success, and women placed greater value than men on balancing professional and personal roles. Women also were more likely to seek and take advantage of the flexibility to work part-time or interrupt their careers temporarily.[14]

Gender and the balancing of work and family responsibilities are just two of the many personal and organizational factors that influence an individual's career path and professional development. Just as each PT must create an individual plan for professional development, each PT construes career success differently. Reflection on the personal meaning of professional competence, professional development, and career success, as well as their interrelationship, may help PTs set meaningful goals.

ORGANIZATIONAL IMPACT ON PROFESSIONAL DEVELOPMENT

Organizations may have a significant impact on professional development. Obviously, one aspect of professional competence is the ability to apply professional knowledge and skills in the organizational setting. However, organizations also may shape professionals through educational offerings and reimbursement for continuing education.

More important, as Smith notes, organizations shape PTs through *organizational socialization,* "the process by which an individual enters an organization and becomes a fully participating and effective member."[16] Socialization is not a discrete event, but rather a continuous, interactive process in which the individual and the organization learn and respond to each other's needs.[16] For the PT, an important part of this process is learning and incorporating the organization's values and culture.

At some point in their career, PTs and other professionals may find their personal or professional values in conflict with the organizational culture and values. When major differences arise between the accepted ethical standards of the profession and the formal or informal ethical stance of the organization, the PT either must try to change the organizational stance or resign. The *Guide for Professional Conduct* states, "A physical therapist shall advise his/her employer(s) of any employer practice that causes a physical therapist to be in conflict with the ethical principles of the association. A physical therapist shall seek to eliminate aspects of his/her employment that are in conflict with the ethical principles of the association" (GPC 4.3B).[3]

FURTHER THOUGHTS

Success or failure in professional development depends on the individual's motivation and enthusiasm. The heart of professional development is a willingness to engage in continual self-assessment and reflection; without these two components, professional development runs the risk of degenerating into simply ensuring minimal competence.

CASE SCENARIOS

Case Scenario 1

You have just been appointed to the Board of Physical Therapy Practice in your state. The first order of business is to respond to the governor's order that each profession present a plan to ensure the continued competence of licensed practitioners in the state.
- *What are your recommendations?*

Case Scenario 2

The hospital system for which you work has decided to capture the market for physical therapy for individuals with lymphedema, and it plans to open a center within 3 months. You have been asked to attend an intensive course on lymphedema management and to become certified in these treatments. You are the organization's last hope; no one else wants to do it.
- *How do you decide whether to comply with the request?*

QUESTIONS FOR REFLECTION

1. What dimensions of professional competence are evaluated by tools used to assess the performance of physical therapy students in clinical affiliations?
2. How should regulatory agencies evaluate professional competence? How should this be done by organizations and individual PTs?
3. The public has become increasingly concerned about incompetent practitioners. What can PTs do to protect the public from incompetent therapists and substandard care? Why do PTs and other professionals fail to report incompetent or impaired colleagues?
4. Describe your approach to professional development. How do you plan and evaluate professional development?
5. Has socialization into your organization enhanced or hindered your professional development?
6. Where would you place yourself on the continuum of novice to expert?
7. What are your indicators for determining career success? What challenges have you encountered in balancing career and personal roles and responsibilities?
8. What would facilitate your commitment to professional development? How will you know your professional development is sufficient? What are your external or internal motivators for professional development and career success?

References

1. Eraut M. *Developing professional knowledge and competence.* London: Falmer; 1994.
2. Rothstein JM. Are you financing a sham? *Phys Ther* 2001;81(9):1500-1501.
3. American Physical Therapy Association. *Guide for Professional Conduct.* Retrieved October 29, 2004, at http://www.apta.org/PT_Practice/ethics_pt/pro_conduct
4. American Physical Therapy Association. *Board of directors statement on professional development.* Retrieved January 9, 2004, at http://www.apta.org/Career_center/career_management/WhatIsProfDev
5. Epstein RM, Hundert EM. Defining and assessing professional competence. *JAMA* 2002:287(2): 226-235.
6. Jensen GM, Gwyer J, Shepard KF, et al. Expert practice in physical therapy. *Phys Ther* 2000;80(1):28-43.
7. Resnik L, Jensen GM. Using clinical outcomes to explore the theory of expert practice in physical therapy. *Phys Ther* 2003;83:1090-1106.
8. Shepard KF, Jensen GM. Physical therapist curricula for the 1990s: Educating the reflective practitioner. *Phys Ther* 1990;70(9):566-573.
9. Schon DA. *Educating the reflective practitioner.* San Francisco: Jossey-Bass; 1987.
10. Gardner DL, Seymour RJ, Lacefield WE. Mandatory continuing education or periodic reexamination? *Phys Ther* 1981;61(7):1029-1034.
11. Paschal KA, Jensen GM, Mostrom E. Building portfolios: A means for developing habits of reflective practice in physical therapy education. *J Phys Ther Educ* 2002;16(3):38-53.
12. Chartered Society of Physiotherapy. *Developing a portfolio: A guide for CSP members.* London: The Society; 2001.
13. *Merriam-Webster Online Dictionary.* Information retrieved January 21, 2004, at http://www.merriam-webster.com
14. Rozier CK, Raymond MJ, Goldstein MS et al. Gender and physical therapy career success factors. *Phys Ther* 1998;78:690-704.
15. Kemp KI, Scholz CA, Sanford TL et al. Salary and status differences between male and female physical therapists. *Phys Ther* 1979;59:1095-1101.
16. Smith DM. Organizational socialization of physical therapists. *Phys Ther* 1989;69(4):282-286.

Future Challenges in Physical Therapy

The physical therapy profession has its roots in rehabilitation of those injured by national calamities, epidemic diseases, and wars. The profession grew out of a national need to alleviate human suffering, and it continues to be recognized for the humanistic qualities of its members. A profession, such as physical therapy, that has been able to mobilize resources in times of national need should be able to respond to this call for research by the year 2005. To do less would betray the physical therapy profession's moral mission, a mission aimed at assisting in the achievement of optimal human function.

— Andrew A. Guccione, E. Mark Goldstein, and Steven Elliott[1]

The future of physical therapy is in your hands. To each mind is offered its choice between ideas and somnolence, its choice between questing and resting. Take whichever you please. You can never have both.

— Helen J. Hislop[2]

The difference between our future and our destiny will be measured in our commitment.

— Steven L. Wolf[3]

PHYSICAL THERAPY'S MORAL MISSION

The practice of physical therapy has undergone dramatic changes since the profession's beginnings in the early twentieth century. These changes have been driven in part by events outside the profession; for example, the discipline of physical therapy was born out of the devastating human consequences of World War I and grew in response to subsequent wars and the polio epidemic of the 1950s. Nevertheless, physical therapy as a profession could not have developed without the vision of its early leaders, who recognized the benefits caring combined with science could offer those with movement disorders. Although the details of the vision may change, the sense of professionalism, which is central to every physical therapist's (PT's) practice, is fundamentally linked to this concept of scientifically informed service to patients with movement dysfunctions.

The purposes of this book were to elaborate on the nature and history of professionalism in physical therapy, describe the professional roles of the PT, examine the practice settings in which PTs work, evaluate the effects of organizational and societal environments on professionalism, discuss professional development, and examine contemporary issues. This final chapter presents a discussion of issues the profession and the individual PTs must face in the future (Box 11-1). The three-realm and four-component models provide a framework for consideration of these important topics.

THE FUTURE IN THREE REALMS

The Individual Realm

Many of the professional issues that arise in the individual realm are related to the managed care system, potential changes with the transition to the doctor of physical therapy (DPT) degree, and PTs' ability to achieve the goal of autonomous practice, which was articulated in the current vision statement, Vision 2020, published by the American Physical Therapy Association (APTA).[4]

PTs report that they are under greater pressure to work efficiently, i.e., increase the number of billable units per unit time, and that they spend much of their remaining time negotiating for reimbursement for individual patients and documenting to justify the care for which they have just negotiated. These demands will continue to increase.

Managed care also has reduced the total time PTs work with patients by limiting the number of visits allowed. Formerly, therapists might work with patients for months and forge strong bonds with them. This is now much less common, and no signs indicate that the pattern will change, either for the better or the worse. This may affect relationships with patients, the primary source of many PTs' professional fulfillment, which in turn may result in increased job dissatisfaction, job-related

---

Box 11-1 **FUTURE ISSUES IN PHYSICAL THERAPY**

1. Effects of managed care on professional relationship with patients
2. Focus on reimbursement
3. Transition to a "doctoring profession"
4. Effective interventions and validated evaluation tools
5. Autonomous practice
6. Impact of technology
7. Scholarship in professionalism and ethics
8. Professional relationship with other PTs and health care professionals
9. Changing role of the PT in society
10. Changing role of the PT in organizations
11. Health care policy and the health care system
12. Effects of physician ownership of a physical therapy practice and self-referral
13. Disparities in available health care resources
14. Disparities in the availability of health care information
15. Increased emphasis on lifestyle-induced diseases
16. Global political issues and international economics
17. Role of complementary therapies
18. Cultural competence
19. Lack of diversity in the physical therapy profession
20. Conflicts between professional ethics and organizational or societal values

stress, and burnout. It remains to be seen how entry-level preparation at the doctoral level will provide PTs with the skills and values to keep the central focus of their practice on relationships formed with patients.

The potential effects of having the DPT as an entry-level degree raises other questions. How will the degree affect PTs' sense of professionalism? For example, will they be more autonomous, more responsible, more caring? PTs who earn the DPT may be more prepared to advocate for their patients at every level, more willing to create *pro bono* networks to help the uninsured, more involved in health and wellness efforts, and more prepared to screen and refer to other health care providers. However, until a critical mass of PTs with the DPT degree exists, we can only speculate on the impact of the degree on the behavior, skills, and values of PTs in their professional relationships with patients and other health care providers. The impact on advancement of the profession is also speculative. What changes might be seen in the APTA's House of Delegates, for example, if all delegates had a DPT degree?

With regard to the practice of physical therapy, most agree that all PTs will engage in evidence-based practice in the future. Nevertheless, some aspects have yet to be determined, such as whether PTs will become users of research, whether they will alter their practice based on current evidence, and whether a handful of researchers can supply the evidence for the entire profession. The law of supply and demand may determine the advancement of an evidence-based foundation; that is, the demand for evidence may need to become more firmly established among PTs to propel the effort required to achieve a truly evidence-based profession. Perhaps the new generation of PTs with the DPT will shoulder this responsibility as a routine component of their practices.

Taking another tack, some health care providers and consumers have become more interested in complementary therapies (e.g., acupuncture, Feldenkrais, Craniosacral, Alexander technique, rolfing, therapeutic touch). Continued interest in these parallel lines of health care seems likely, and some insurers may provide menus of benefits that allow consumers to choose alternatives to traditional medicine. However, the APTA points out that the effectiveness and efficacy of such techniques need to be established before their widespread endorsement by PTs and their use in daily practice.[5]

With greater autonomy, the PT can more easily incorporate critical inquiry and the various roles of the physical therapist—other elements of the individual realm—into daily practice. Although the number of states that allow direct access has increased, the number of PTs engaged in primary practice appears to be relatively small, and the roles of PTs and their career ladders remain relatively unchanged. The next few decades may find more PTs working in primary practice and having more professional autonomy; they may then be able to move more easily into the other roles of the PT. For example, PTs may choose to pursue alternative financial arrangements with patients, such as sliding-scale private payment, as they follow patients who are in the health care system from its fringes, which may be the truest form of autonomy. These types of niche practices would contrast with current and past arrangements, which have focused on serving those with third-party reimbursement. Of course, if all PTs were to practice that independently, the impact on the professional association would be dramatic.

Another major influence on the future will be the impact of technology both in and beyond health care. Many patients have as much access to information as their health care providers, and the use of technological interventions to assist in patient education, adherence, prevention, and intervention in movement disorders is limited only by the imagination. Electronic transmission of documentation and reimbursement systems is already commonly assumed. With technological resources, the challenge for PTs will be to bridge the gap between the "haves" and the "have nots." Some consumers will be able to use computers and other technological devices to keep informed about health care, but others will lack any type of access to this information. Technology may prove to be one of the major cultural gaps, especially in health care.

Evaluating the changes in the professional role over time will be difficult because relatively little scholarship has been devoted to professionalism and ethics in physical therapy. A number of authors have noted that greater autonomy will increase the complexity of professional and ethical problems.[6-10] Therefore, as PTs practice in more autonomous roles, the need for scholarship in the areas of ethics and professionalism will increase. For example, relatively little is known about how PTs see their professional role or about relationships with patients. Without descriptive and qualitative studies, it will be difficult to determine the true impact of the movement toward a doctoring profession. Similarly, further scholarship is needed to identify emerging ethical issues in physical therapy. Triezenberg's[11] 1996 study involving ethics experts delineated a number of future ethical issues: (1) environmental issues and hazards, (2) discrimination in employment, (2) reporting of misconduct by colleagues, (3) limits of personal relationships, (4) encroachment of other disciplines, (5) use of interventions without research validation, (6) advertisement of physical therapy services, and (7) physical and sexual abuse of patients.

The Institutional Realm

The individual concerns of PTs will be viewed through a different lens in the institutional, or organizational, realm, resulting in a different interpretation of these issues. The role of the PT in organizations and the potential conflict between PTs' professional values and those of the organization will continue to evolve. Managed care has pressured health care organizations to remain profitable. This has caused some organizations to adopt policies for increasing productivity that conflict with the professional values of physical therapy. These types of conflicts are particularly stressful when jobs are less plentiful. In the future, PTs will need organizational skills that allow them to negotiate such conflicts successfully and enable them to contribute to the development of more effective organizational structures, perhaps beyond the model of traditional health care systems. Many PTs are already working in contractual or *per diem* positions rather than traditional employee-employer work relationships. The shift in health care expenditures to individuals with chronic conditions provides PTs with opportunities to create new models of care; this type of care would reduce and eliminate the movement dysfunctions inherent in many chronic conditions while incorporating a broader concept of health and wellness that reaches beyond traditional "health" care.

The response of hospitals and other health care organizations to the change in the entry-level degree and to PTs' efforts to achieve autonomous practice cannot yet be gauged. In the more hierarchical, bureaucratic organizations, changes in relative power and status are likely to occur slowly, if at all. Organizational change is critical for meeting the goals the profession has established. For example, even in states with direct access, organizational policies often require a physician's referral. Therefore if PTs are to become autonomous practitioners, alternatives to traditional health care organizations may need to be identified.

Without organizational support and a transformation of organizational culture to promote professional autonomy, PTs will find it difficult to practice patient-focused, evidence-based care. The issue is whether the organizational health care culture will adapt to allow all health care professionals to generate evidence, have easy access to the evidence, and participate in interdisciplinary guidelines for care based on the evidence. An increasingly important organizational concern may be what to do if two professional groups produce conflicting evidence.

Some argue that, because organizations are so difficult to change, the real solution lies in PTs owning or controlling more physical therapy practice settings. This would require more private practices and also more PTs willing to advance to higher levels of management in existing health care organizations. At the same time, many are worried about the fate of hospital-based physical therapy services. These may not be considered core services as hospitals, bearing the financial burden of providing care to the uninsured and underinsured, seek to streamline their operations.

PTs may also be challenged by the competition among providers that has been fostered by managed care. This environment has had a stifling effect on teamwork, the basic unit of learning organizations and a critical factor in the treatment of complex patient problems. It also affects professional relationships among PTs at competing institutions in a community. Sharing of information may be discouraged in an effort to demonstrate loyalty to the employer and to maintain a competitive advantage.

Little is known about the PT as organizational citizen. Because of the lack of a research baseline, predicting changes in the role of the PT in health care organizations is difficult; more scholarship in this area obviously is needed.

The Societal Realm

Managed care has provided a powerful lesson in the importance of societal-level issues. Changes in Medicare and other health insurance reimbursement have had a profound effect in almost every area of daily physical therapy practice. National and state health care policies, such as the Health Insurance Portability and Accountability Act, have also had an impact.

At one time few people had any concept of a PT's roles. As PTs move to embrace the issues of health, wellness, and prevention, they must find ways to communicate this evolving role to individual consumers, state regulatory boards, legislators, patients' associations, and other professionals. This will become particularly important as health care policy continues to shape reimbursement and health care delivery methods. Involvement in the political process will continue to be important for PTs. As professionals, PTs have an obligation to evaluate health care policy not only from the perspective of reimbursement and self-interest but also for its effect on patients. Effective engagement in the political process requires partnering with patients, consumer groups, and other health care providers with the goal of developing a good and fair health care system. This is particularly important in light of the increasing criticism of professionals in the United States (see Chapter 1). Health care disparities, access to health care, and equitable financing remain critical challenges to PTs as professionals and as citizens.

Legislation also directly affects the model of physical therapy practice. For instance, laws allowing physician ownership of physical therapy services have led to concerns about the ability of independent physical therapy practices to survive. The dominance of physician-owned outpatient services and the resurgence of physician self-referral could have a negative effect on the practice of physical therapy unless alternative models of practice are identified and PTs are prepared to manage them. The effect of legislation on patient choice, the control of practice quality, the potential decrease in hospital-based PT services, and the autonomy of PTs directly employed by physicians will require close monitoring.

As a national representative organization of PTs, the APTA has the opportunity to influence all three realms of physical therapy practice. Membership in the organization provides resources, influence, and clout that may not be available to the individual PT. Although individual PTs can influence health legislation by writing their legislators, the APTA represents ten of thousands of individuals in its lobbying efforts. Unfortunately, the percentage of PTs who are members of the APTA has been declining in recent years. An individual PT obviously will not agree with every position taken by the association, but those who choose not to be members sacrifice opportunities to influence the practice of physical therapy in all three realms.

The broadest level of societal perspective is global. The increased interaction and sharing of ideas and resources made possible by the Internet and other technological advances are exciting opportunities. This potential for communication enriches PTs' professional experiences as they seek to resolve issues in all three realms. The ability to compare and contrast multiple models of the three realms is profoundly important to PTs striving individually and collectively to meet their professional responsibilities.

PROFESSIONALISM AND THE PHYSICAL THERAPIST

A Framework for Considering Professional Problems

The professionalism of PTs has been shaped not only by historical events but also by the moral commitment of individual PTs. Each generation of PTs has encountered unanticipated challenges that required new professional skills, knowledge, and behavior. The four-component model of professional behavior provides a framework for analyzing professional issues and for developing appropriate strategies for dealing deal with those issues.[12,13] According to this model, professional behavior involves four overlapping processes: professional sensitivity, professional judgment, professional motivation, and professional conduct or courage (Table 11-1).

Table 11-1 | **Four-Component Model of Professional Behavior**

Component	Elements
Professional sensitivity	Recognition of professional issues, problems, and situations; ability to interpret professional situations and project consequences of alternative actions
Professional judgment	Ability to make appropriate professional decisions based on professional norms and standards and society's legitimate expectations of professional behavior
Professional motivation	Ability to prioritize professional values appropriately in relation to personal, clinical, organizational, or other values
Professional conduct or courage	Ability to implement professional judgment, derived from character, implementation skills, and specific contextual knowledge

Modified from Baldwin DC Jr, Bunch WH. Moral reasoning, professionalism, and the teaching of ethics to orthopaedic surgeons. Clin Orthop 2000;378:97-103.

To illustrate how this framework might help in analyzing a professional problem, we might consider breaches of confidentiality. Consider the example of two PTs who are discussing the progress of a celebrity patient while they are riding in an elevator. This unintentional lapse might be contrasted to the lapse that might be involved if a PT were to respond to a reporter's telephone inquiry regarding the celebrity patient's progress. Whereas the first example most likely represents a failure in professional sensitivity, the second is more likely poor professional judgement. One can imagine different strategies from the three realms to address these issues. Individual health care providers can provide guidance to each other in such situations. For instance, a simple reminder about the public setting to those conversing on the elevator would be effective. In the organizational realm, institutions may present inservices to remind PTs of their professional obligations, reinforcing moral motivation.

CONCLUSION

This text has explored the many dimensions of professionalism in physical therapy—roles, setting, self-concept, environments, and development. Becoming a professional is a journey, and each physical therapist travels a slightly different path toward the common goal. The journeys of generations of physical therapists are the collective history that points to the future. The profession undoubtedly will continue to be shaped by its history; at the same time, its future depends on the decisions, actions, and commitment of each physical therapist.

CASE SCENARIO

Case Scenario 1

You have been appointed to a strategic planning committee of the APTA. Your task is to determine the top three issues facing the profession and to formulate a strategic plan (see Chapter 9) for achieving goals related to these issues.
- *Use the (strengths, weaknesses, opportunities, and threats (SWOT) format for your strategic plan. Figure 11-1 guides you in your SWOT analysis and in developing a plan.*

QUESTIONS FOR REFLECTION

1. Make your own list of the top 10 future professional issues in physical therapy. Have you chosen issues that are not included in Box 11-1? If so, provide rationales for them.
2. What are the five most important issues facing you as an individual professional? Use Figure 11-1 to develop a plan to achieve five goals related to these five issues (one for each of the five roles of the physical therapist).
3. Go to the APTA's web site. How would you characterize the membership? What effect do you think the lack of diversity in the membership has on the organization and the profession? What could be done to improve this situation?
4. What are the advantages and disadvantages of belonging to the APTA? Some argue that not belonging to the APTA is "getting a free ride" because nonmembers

SWOT Analysis

Top three professional issues facing physical therapy

1. _____

2. _____

3. _____

Goals related to the top three issues

1. _____

2. _____

3. _____

Strengths
What are the strengths of the profession that will help in achieving these goals?

_____

_____

_____

_____

Weaknesses
What are the weaknesses of the profession that may hinder the effort to achieve these goals?

_____

_____

_____

Opportunities
What are the internal and external environmental factors that you capitalize upon to achieve your goal?
(Be sure to include organizational and social environments)

_____

_____

_____

Threats
What are the internal and external environmental factors that could jeopardize achievement of your goal?
(Be sure to include organizational and social environments)

_____

_____

_____

Plan
Outline a plan to achieve your goals. This should include a timeline, delineation of roles and responsibilities
of particular groups and individuals, and a plan for measuring whether the goal has been achieved.

_____

_____

_____

_____

_____

_____

_____

Figure 11-1. SWOT analysis.

benefit from resources provided by members. Do you agree? What could be done to increase the percentage of physical therapists who are members?

5. Reimbursement plays a major role in physical therapy. In fact, some would argue that too much emphasis is placed on reimbursement. Professional organizations have been criticized for being self-serving special interest groups. From this perspective, it could be argued that the APTA should analyze health care policies primarily for fairness and access of disadvantaged populations and not merely for their effect on reimbursement of physical therapy services. As professionals, physical therapists have responsibilities to society. Do the societal obligations of professionals extend to the activity of professional associations? If so, what should the APTA do to meet these obligations?

REFERENCES

1. Guccione AA, Goldstein M, Elliott S. Clinical research agenda for physical therapy. *Phys Ther* 2000;80:499-513.

2. Hislop HJ. Tenth Mary McMillan Lecture: The not-so-impossible dream. *Phys Ther* 1975;55: 1069-1080.

3. Wolf SL. Thirty-third Mary McMillan Lecture: Look forward, walk tall: Exploring our "what if" questions. *Phys Ther* 2002;82:1108-1119.

4. American Physical Therapy Association. *APTA vision sentence and vision statement for physical therapy 2020* [HOD 06-00-24-35]. Available from: http://www.apta.org/About/aptamissiongoals/ visionstatement

5. American Physical Therapy Association. *Frequently asked practice questions*. Retrieved October 29, 2004 at http://www.apta.org/PT_Practice/FAQ

6. Magistro CM. Clinical decision making in physical therapy: A practitioner's perspective. *Phys Ther* 1989;69:525-534.

7. Singleton MC. Independent practice—on the horns of a dilemma: A special communication. *Phys Ther* 1987;67:54-57.

8. Purtilo RB. Understanding ethical issues: The physical therapist as ethicist. *Phys Ther* 1974;54: 239-242.

9. Purtilo RB. Ethics teaching in allied health fields. *Hastings Cent Rep* 1978;8(2):14-16.

10. Guccione AA. Ethical issues in physical therapy practice: A survey of physical therapists in New England. *Phys Ther* 1980;60:1264-1272.

11. Triezenberg HL. The identification of ethical issues in physical therapy practice. *Phys Ther* 1996;76:1097-1107.

12. Baldwin DC Jr, Bunch WH. Moral reasoning, professionalism, and the teaching of ethics to orthopaedic surgeons. *Clin Orthop* 2000;378:97-103.

13. Rest JR. Background: Theory and research. In Rest JR, Narvaez D, editors. *Moral development in the professions: Psychology and applied ethics*. Hillsdale, NJ: Erlbaum; 1994.

Index

A

Academic coordinator of clinical education (ACCE), 137b
Academic integrity, 145
Academic teaching opportunities, 138-140
Accountability of professionals, 9-12
Achievement, professional, evaluators of, 203-204
Administration
  physical therapy
    contemporary, 151, 154
    history of, 149-151
  physical therapy service, APTA Standards of Practice, 219-222
Advancement of career, 204-205
American Board of Physical Therapy Specialties (ABPTS), 49b
American Physical Therapy Association. *See* APTA
American Women's Physical Therapeutic Association (AWPTA), 27, 34b
Andragogy, 141t-142t
APTA
  clinical research agenda, 112b
  code of ethics
    for consultants, 103-105
    in critical inquiry, 122
  development of, 27, 32
  goals of, 34b
  headquarters, organizational chart for, 156f
  lobbying by, 67-68
  Mary McMillan lectures, 38t-41t
  organizational chart for, 155f
  political action committees, 66-67
  position on autonomous practice, 7b
  statement on professional development, 195b
  vision for future, 45, 88-89

APTA Standards of Practice
  administration of physical therapy service, 219-222
  community responsibility, 225
  education, 224-225
  legal/ethical considerations, 219
  provision of services, 222-224
  research, 225
Arthritis, effectiveness and efficacy studies comparison, 115b
Autonomy
  in decision making, 5-8
  in future of physical therapy, 211
  in patient/client management, 86-87

B

Behavior, professional, four-component model of, 214t
Behaviorism, 141t-142t
Billing for physical therapy services, 159, 161
Biopsychosocial model (Steiner et al.), 72-73
Board certification of specialists, 48-51
Brackett, Elliott, 32
Budget responsibilities of first-line management, 168, 170
Bureaucracy, professional, leadership tasks in, 184b
Business building
  consulting fees, 97-98
  consulting process, 99-100
  skills of good consultant, 100
  trust in consultant/client relationship, 101

C

Cardiovascular pulmonary practice pattern, 61b-62b
Career advancement, 204-205
Case law, affecting higher education, 144t
Case reports, publication of, 117-118
Center coordinator of clinical education (CCCE), 135-136

Page numbers followed by f indicate figures; t, tables; b, boxes.

Certified clinical specialists, distribution
    (in 2003), 50t
Client needs, met by physical therapy
    consultants, 96t
Clinical decision making
    critical inquiry and, 116b
    diagnosis as, 72-73
    in patient/client management process,
        79-81
Clinical expertise, 111
    dimensions of, 197f
Clinical Performance Instrument (CPI), 136
Clinical reasoning, of expert and average
    PTs, 198t
Clinical research
    agenda (APTA), 112b
    collaboration on, 120
    networks, 113b
Code of ethics
    in administration role of PTs, 174
    for consultants, 103
    in critical inquiry, 122
    regarding education, 144
Cognitivism, 141t-142t
Collaboration, on clinical research, 120
Commercial model of professionalism, 10
Commission on Accreditation of Physical
    Therapy Education (CAPTE), 116,
    130, 139
Community responsibility, APTA Standards
    of Practice, 225
Competence
    continuing, 145
    and professional development,
        evaluation of, 200-202
    scope of, 194-196
Complex adaptive system for health care,
    183-184
Components of practice patterns, 63t
Computer-based documentation, 165
Conflict of interest
    administrator's role and, 175-176
    in patient/client management, 88
Constructivism, 141t-142t
Consultant/client relationship, trust in,
    101
Consultation
    consulting fees, 97-98
    consulting process, 99-100
    ethical and legal issues in, 101-105

Consultation (Continued)
    physical therapy, 93-97
    services provided by physical therapists, 95b
    skills of good consultant, 100
Consulting agreement, components of, 103b
Continuing education
    mandatory, 200-201, 200t
    quality of, 199-200
    teaching opportunities in, 137-138
Contract law, 102-103
Control, exercised at different management
    levels, 158t
CPT codes, 160b-161b
Critical inquiry
    criteria for, 116b
    ethical and legal issues in, 122-125
    history of, 109-111
    staff PT roles in, 117-122
Cultural competence
    applied to organizations, 187
    evaluation of, 187-188
    individual, 186
    levels of, 188t
Curriculum, physical therapy, first
    recommended, 131b
Curriculum requirements, PTA programs,
    58b-59b

D

Decision making
    autonomy in, 5-8
    clinical
        critical inquiry and, 116b
        diagnosis as, 72-73
        in patient/client management process,
            79-81
Delegation
    of duties to PTAs, 56-57, 59
    and supervision of support personnel,
        166-168
Development of values
    ethical issues, 35
    professional recognition, 36
Diagnosis
    as clinical decision making, 72-73
    as end product of evaluation, 71
Diagnosis-related groups (DRGs), 76-77
Direct access
    perspective of the practitioner, 53-54
    perspective of the profession, 51-53

Director of clinical education (DCE), 137b
Disablement model, 62-64
Discharge planning, 74-78
Discontinuance of care, 75b, 78-79
Doctorate in physical therapy (DPT), 7-8
    future of, 211
    perspective of the practitioner, 47-48
    perspective of the profession, 46-47
    rationale for awarding, 12-13
Documentation
    APTA Standards of Practice, 224
    computer-based, 165
    correct and incorrect, 162t-163t
    defined, 161
    general rules of, 164b-165b
    medical record, 163

E

Education
    APTA Standards of Practice, 224-225
    of client, health risk discussion points
        for, 67b
    clinical, teaching opportunities in, 135-137
    continuing
        mandatory, 200-201, 200t
        quality of, 199-200
        teaching opportunities in, 137-138
    physical therapy
        ethical and legal issues in, 140, 144-145
        history of, 129-132
    professional, theories of teaching and
        learning in, 140
Educational roles of physical therapist
    academic teaching opportunities, 138-140
    forms of teaching opportunities, 132-133
    instruction of patients, 133
    making presentations, 133-134
    teaching opportunities
        in clinical education, 135-137
        in continuing education, 137-138
Effectiveness study, comparison with efficacy
    study, 115b
Employment, legal status of, 102
Episode of physical therapy prevention, 65
Equipment lists for 1932 and 1999, 83b
Ethical issues
    in administration role of PTs, 174-176
    in consultation, 101-105
    in critical inquiry, 122-125
    development of, 35

Ethical issues (*Continued*)
    in patient/client management, 85-89
    in physical therapy education, 140,
        144-145
Ethical principles of human research, 123b
Ethical standards, self-regulation of, 8-9
Ethics literature
    administrator's role in, 176
    critical inquiry role in, 125
    and educator's role, 145
    peer-reviewed, 88-89
Evaluation
    diagnosis as end product of, 71
    of professional achievement, 203-204
Evidence-based medicine (EBM), 111-114,
    124-125
Evolution of physical therapy
    physical therapy today, 34-35
    pioneers of physical therapy, 32-33
    social history, 24-32
Expertise
    attributes of expert and average PTs, 198t
    in continuum of professional development,
        196-197

F

Faculty, clinical physical therapy: criteria
    for, 135b
Familiar-to-unfamiliar decision continuum,
    79-80
Fee setting for consulting, 98b
Fidelity, managed care and, 88
Financial responsibilities in physical
    therapy, 157t
First-line management
    budget responsibilities, 168, 170
    human resources responsibilities, 171
    information responsibilities, 171-173
    operations responsibilities, 171
Foundation for Physical Therapy, 111b
Functions of professional organization, 23

G

Gender differences in career advancement,
    204-205
Goal-driven portfolio, 202
Goals of AWPTA and APTA, 34b
Goldthwait, Joel, 32
Gorgas, Major General William, 32
Granger, Frank, 32

Guide for Professional Conduct, 85-87
  in administration role of PTs, 174-175
  for consultants, 103-105
  in critical inquiry, 122
  regarding education, 144
Guide to Physical Therapist Practice, 59-66
  broadening of practice context, 64-66
  perspective of the practitioner, 66
  perspective of the profession, 60
  practice patterns, 61-64
Guidelines for critiquing research
    reports, 118b
Guild model of professionalism, 10-11

H

Health care
  cultural competence in organizations, 187
  evaluating cultural competence,
    187-188
  future of
    individual realm, 210-212
    institutional realm, 212-213
    societal realm, 213-214
  individual cultural competence, 186
  international realm, 189
  realms of, 184-186
Health care costs
  legislation to control, 27
  and referral relationships, 82
Health care system
  and autonomous practice, 8
  complexity of, 182-184
  trend toward product-line
    management, 151
Health Insurance Portability and
    Accountability Act (HIPPA), 172b
Health risk discussion points for client
    education, 67b
History
  of critical inquiry, 109-111
  of development of PTAs, 55-56
  of physical therapy administration,
    149-151
  of physical therapy education, 129-132
  social, of physical therapy, 24-32
Hooked on Evidence, 113b
Human research, ethical principles of, 123b
Human resources responsibilities
  of first-line management, 171
  in physical therapy, 157t

Human subjects, protection of, 122-123
Hypothesis-oriented algorithm for clinicians
    (HOAC), 72, 74

I

Identity periods (Purtilo), 35
Individual cultural competence, 186
Individual professionalism, 2, 15-16
Individual realm of health care, 184-186
  future of, 210-212
Information mastery, comparison with
    traditional EBP, 115f
Information responsibilities
  of first-line management, 171-173
  in physical therapy, 157t
Informed consent
  APTA Standards of Practice, 222
  in patient/client management, 87-88
Institutional realm of health care,
    184-186
  future of, 212-213
Institutional review boards, 123-124
Instruction of patients, 133
Integrity, academic, 145
Integumentary practice pattern, 61b
Interactive model of professionalism,
    11-12
International realm of health care, 189
Internet, database sources of evidence
    for practice, 114b
Interpersonal relationships, in patient/
    client management, 83-84
Intervention
  APTA Standards of Practice, 223
  discharge/discontinuation of, 224
  instructional, plan of care with, 133b

K

Knowledge base of expert and average
    PTs, 198t

L

Leadership
  physical therapy and, 188
  tasks, in complex adaptive system, 184b
  theories, 152t-153t, 173
Learning objectives
  ABCD method of writing, 143b
  taxonomy of, 143b
Learning theories, 141t-142t

Legal issues
    in administration role of PTs, 174-176
    in consultation, 101-105
    in critical inquiry, 122-125
    in patient/client management, 85-89
    in physical therapy education, 140, 144-145
Legislation
    affecting direct access, 52t
    effect on physical therapy practice, 213
Literature
    ethics
        administrator's role in, 176
        critical inquiry role in, 125
        and educator's role, 145
        peer-reviewed, 88-89
    professionalism as described in, 13b, 14b
Lobbying, by APTA, 67-68

M

Managed care
    cost minimization by, 182-183
    and fidelity, 88
    impact on concept of profession, 6
    societal realm, 213-214
Management, first-line, 168-173
Management theories, 152t-153t
Mandatory continuing education,
        200-201, 200t
Matrix method of reviewing research
        studies, 119f
McMillan, Mary, 32-33
    APTA lecture series, 38t-41t
Medicare
    memorandum on discharge planning,
        76b
    Part B, rules for student provision of
        services, 136b
    supervision requirements for PTAs, 169t
Medicine, evidence-based (EBM),
        111-114
Midlevel managers and CEOs, responsibilities
        of, 173
Milestones in history of physical therapy,
        25t-26t, 28t-29t
Mission statement, 203
Models of professionalism, 10-12
Moral mission of physical therapy,
        209-210
Musculoskeletal practice pattern,
        61b-62b

N

Needs-based consultation, 95b
Neuromuscular practice pattern, 61b-62b
New concepts and technology, assessment
        of, 120-121

O

Oath
    correlated with principles of code of
        ethics, 17b-18b
    in physical therapy, 15
Obligations of professional organization, 23
Occupation to profession continuum, 5f
Operations responsibilities
    of first-line management, 171
    in physical therapy, 157t
Organizational chart
    for APTA, 155f
    for APTA headquarters, 156f
Organizational ethics, 175
Organizational impact on professional
        development, 205
Organizational terminology, 183t
Organizational theories, 152t-153t
Outcome competencies, APTA-developed, 48
Outcomes
    addressed in patient/client management
        process, 79
    research, 114-115
Ozar's models of professionalism, 11t

P

Participation Method Assessment
        Instrument (PMAI), 85b
Patient abandonment, 78-79
Patient/client management
    billing for physical therapy services,
        159, 161
    clinical decision making, 79-81
    comparison with consulting process, 99f
    delegation and supervision of support
        personnel, 166-168
    discharge planning and discontinuance
        of care, 74-79
    documentation, 161-165
    ethical and legal issues, 85-89
    evaluation and diagnosis, 71-73
    interpersonal relationships, 83-84
    outcomes, 79
    professional managerial issues, 154

Patient/client management (*Continued*)
prognosis, 73-74
referral relationships, 81-82
technological advances, 82-83
Patient-focused identity period, 35
Patients
cultural evaluation of, 189b
instruction of, 133
Payer mix, sample budget with, 170f
Peer review, 200t, 201-202
Peer-reviewed ethics literature, 88-89
Physiatrists, 33
Physical therapist assistants
creation of position of, 27
history of, 55-56
Medicare supervision requirements
for, 169t
perspective of
the practitioner, 57, 59
the profession, 54-55
recent studies on, 56-57
Physical therapists
accountability of, 9-12
autonomy in decision making, 5-8
consultation services provided by, 95b
CPT codes used by, 160b-161b
direct access issue, 51-54
educational roles of, 132-140
framework for considering professional
problems, 214-215
perspective on
board certification, 50-51
DPTs, 47-48
PTAs, 57, 59
risk reduction/prevention role, 66
roles in critical inquiry, 117-122
self-regulation of ethical standards, 8-9
Physical therapy
administration
contemporary, 151, 154
history of, 149-151
and concepts of professionalism, 12-15
consultation, 93-97
control exercised at different management
levels in, 158t
doctorate in. *See* Doctorate in physical
therapy (DPT)
education
ethical and legal issues in, 140, 144-145
history of, 129-132

Physical therapy (*Continued*)
ethics positions in, 37t
evolution
physical therapy today, 34-35
pioneers of physical therapy, 32-33
social history, 24-32
Foundation for, 111b
future issues in, 210b
international realm of, 189
leadership and, 188
levels of management and
responsibilities in, 157t
moral mission of, 209-210
Ozar's models of professionalism
applied to, 11t
practice patterns, 61-64
professional perspective on
board certification of specialists, 49-50
direct access issue, 51-53
*Guide to Physical Therapist
Practice,* 60
PTAs, 54-55
successful treatment, factors
important to, 86b
use of PMAI in, 85b
World Confederation for (WCPT), 37,
42t, 43
Physical therapy diagnosis, 71-72
Physician-owned physical therapy
services, 82
Plan of care
APTA Standards of Practice, 223
components of, 73-74
with instructional interventions, 133b
Political action committees (PACs), 66-67
Portfolio
compilation of, 200t, 202
goal-driven, 202
Power approach to professions in general, 4-5
Practice
database sources of evidence for, 114b
evidence-based (EBP), 111-114
ethics and, 124-125
Practice patterns of physical therapy, 61-64
Practice style of expert and average
PTs, 198t
Presentations, educational, 133-134
Prevention of illness
services geared to, 65
types of, 64

Processual approach to professions in
general, 3-4
Productivity expectations, survey of, 171t
Products and courses, questions for
assessing, 121b
Professional development
activities promoting, 198-200
and competence, evaluation of, 200-202
organizational impact on, 205
planning
goal-driven portfolio, 202
process of reflection and, 203
Professional development continuum
expertise, 196-197, 198t
quality, 196
scope of competence, 194-196
Professional recognition, 36
Professionalism
commercial model of, 10
framework for considering professional
problems, 214-215
individual, 2, 15-16
physical therapy and, 12-15
Professionalization, shared history as
key to, 23-24
Professions
accountability of professionals, 9-12
autonomy, 5-8
characteristics of, 4b
power approach, 4-5
preliminary definitions of, 2
processual approach, 3-4
self-regulation of ethical standards, 8-9
sociological perspective, 2-3
structural approach, 3
Prognosis, documented in plan of care,
73-74
PTAs. *See* Physical therapist assistants
PTs. *See* Physical therapists

Q

Quality, in continuum of professional
development, 196

R

Reasoning, clinical, of expert and average
PTs, 198t
Reconstruction Aide Corps, 32-33
Referral relationships, in patient/client
management, 81-82

Reflective knowledge, 198-199
Rehabilitation problem-solving form, 72-73
Relationship-based consultation, 95b
Relicensure, 200t, 201
Request for proposal (RFP) process, 97-98
Research
application and critique of, 117
APTA Standards of Practice, 225
clinical
collaboration on, 120
responsibilities of researchers, 124
reports, guidelines for critiquing, 118b
subject, serving as, 122
who is responsible for, 116
Research networks, clinical, 113b
Review boards, institutional, 123-124

S

Sanderson, Marguerite, 32
Scholarship categories, 139
Schools of physical therapy, first
approved, 132b
Scope of competence, 194-196
Scope of physical therapy practice, 63f, 65f
Self-employed contractor status, comparison
with employee status, 102b
Self-identity period, 35
Self-referral, physician, 82
Self-regulation of ethical standards, 8-9
Service responsibilities
APTA Standards of Practice, 222-224
internal and external, 139
Service-based consultation, 95b
Services, billing for, 159, 161
Shared history, as key to professionalization,
23-24
Skills
of good consultant, 100
lifelong enhancement of, 193-194
Social history of physical therapy, 24-32
Societal identity period, 35
Societal realm of health care, 184-186
future of, 213-214
Sociological perspective on professions in
general, 2-3
Specialists, board certification of, 48-51
Standardized-to-open decision continuum,
79-80
Stark II law, 82
Steps in applying EBM, 113b

Strengths, weaknesses, opportunities, and threats (SWOT), 216f
Structural approach to professions in general, 3
Students, vulnerability of, 145
Studies on PTAs, 56-57
Subjects
  human, protection of, 122-123
  vs. patients, 124
  research, serving as, 122
Supervision of support personnel, 166-168
Support personnel, delegation and supervision of, 166-168

T

Teaching opportunities
  academic, 138-140
  in clinical education, 135-137
  in continuing education, 137-138
Technological advances, affecting patient/client management, 82-83
Technology
  in future of physical therapy, 211-212
  and new concepts, assessment of, 120-121

Theories of organization, management, and leadership, 152t-153t
Theories of teaching and learning in professional education, 140
Tips for giving good presentations, 134b
Transfer or referral, Medicare memorandum on, 76b
Transition DPT programs, 48
Trust, in consultant/client relationship, 101
Trust-based consultation, 95b

V

Values
  development of, 35-37
  of expert and average PTs, 198t
Vision for the future, APTA, 45, 88-89

W

Whistleblowing, 176
WHO model, 72
World Confederation for Physical Therapy (WCPT), 37, 42t, 43